Easy

H CLOSE TO
ome

NEW YORK CITY

including
Nearby New York and Nearby New Jersey

CHRISTOPHER BROOKS
AND
CATHERINE BROOKS

MENASHA RIDGE PRESS
Birmingham, Alabama

Easy Hikes Close to Home: New York City

Published by Menasha Ridge Press
Distributed by Publishers Group West
First edition, first printing

ISBN 978-0-89732-892-0

Cover by Scott McGrew
Cover photo (Hook Mountain State Park) by Christopher and Catherine Brooks
All interior photos by Christopher and Catherine Brooks
Text design by Annie Long
Maps by Christopher and Catherine Brooks

Menasha Ridge Press
P.O. Box 43673
Birmingham, AL 35243
www.menasharidge.com

This book is meant only as a guide to select trails in the New York City area
and does not guarantee hiker safety in any way—you hike at your own risk.
Neither Menasha Ridge Press nor Christopher or Catherine Brooks is liable
in any way for property loss or damage, personal injury, or death that result
from accessing or hiking the trails described in the following pages. Please be
aware that hikers have been injured in the New York City area. Be especially
cautious when walking on or near boulders, steep inclines, and drop-offs, and
do not attempt to explore terrain that may be beyond your abilities. To help
ensure an uneventful hike, please read carefully the introduction to this book,
and perhaps get further safety information and guidance from other sources.
Familiarize yourself thoroughly with the areas you intend to visit before
venturing out. Ask questions, and prepare for the unforeseen. Familiarize
yourself with current weather reports, maps of the area you intend to visit,
and any relevant park regulations.

Contents

4   **ABOUT THE AUTHORS**

5   **INTRODUCTION**

7   **TRAIL RECOMMENDATIONS**

9   **MANHATTAN AND PROXIMITY**

10   **Hike 1**: Central Park North Woods Walk
14   **Hike 2**: Clay Pit Ponds Connector
18   **Hike 3**: Governors Island History Hike
23   **Hike 4**: Great Kills Crooke's Point Labyrinth
26   **Hike 5**: High Line Southern Section
30   **Hike 6**: Inwood Hill Park Grand Tour
35   **Hike 7**: Jamaica Bay West Pond Trail
39   **Hike 8**: Pelham Bay Islands Loop

43   **NEARBY NEW YORK**

44   **Hike 9**:   High Tor
47   **Hike 10**: Hook Mountain Challenger
52   **Hike 11**: Muttontown Mystery Trail
57   **Hike 12**: Rockefeller Swan Lake Circuit
60   **Hike 13**: Tallman Hudson River Overlook Trail
64   **Hike 14**: Teatown Triple
69   **Hike 15**: Walt Whitman Sampler

74   **NEARBY NEW JERSEY**

75   **Hike 16**: Cheesequake Natural Area Trail
80   **Hike 17**: High Mountain Summit Loop
85   **Hike 18**: Norvin Green's High Point
89   **Hike 19**: Ramapo Lake Ramble
93   **Hike 20**: Watchung Sierra Sampler

About the Authors

Christopher Brooks

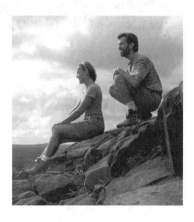

Christopher brings to *Easy Hikes Close to Home: New York City* nearly 30 years of writing experience. An erstwhile editor at *Market Watch* and *Country Living* magazines, he has also contributed to *Family Circle,* the *Christian Science Monitor, Cigar Aficionado,* the *Chicago Tribune,* the *International Herald Tribune,* *USA Today,* and *Diversion.* Christopher, a graduate of Wesleyan University, also writes food-related stories for the *New York Times.*

Catherine Brooks

Catherine Brooks, née Van der Maat, grew up in Belgium. Her enjoyment of nature translates into a fascination with birding, mycology, geology, and botany. Catherine graduated from university as an interpreter before directing marketing for a United States–based multinational corporation.

Together, the Brookses wrote *60 Hikes within 60 Miles: New York City,* which features a great number of easy hikes, as well as more-physical, all-day excursions. They authored the California half of *The Unofficial Guide to the Best RV and Tent Campgrounds in California and the West,* and are also contributors to *Backpacker* magazine. In their free time, Chris and Catherine have hiked the Appalachian Trail, New York's Long Path, the Highlands Trail, the Pacific Crest Trail, the Inca Trail, and most of Connecticut's blue trails.

Introduction

Welcome to *Easy Hikes Close to Home: New York City.* This title in the Easy Hikes series is divided into three Greater New York regions: Manhattan and proximity; nearby New York; and nearby New Jersey.

Numbered map icons on the inside front cover identify each primary trailhead and are keyed to the table of contents and narrative text for each trail. On the inside back cover, a map legend defines symbols for parking, restrooms, trail features, and other details. Armed with this handy guidebook, you can quickly head out the door and, well, take a hike!

Overview

Mileage shown for each hike corresponds to the total distance from start to finish, for loops, out-and-backs, figure-eights, or a combination of shapes. You can shorten or extend many of them with connecting trails.

Trail Maps

Maps for each hike include GPS coordinates. Based on data downloaded from the authors' handheld GPS unit and plotted onto a digital U.S. Geological Survey (USGS) topo map, the coordinates are shown in two formats—as latitude and longitude, and as UTM (Universal Transverse Mercator) coordinates (NAD27).

HIKING ESSENTIALS

Boots should be your footwear of choice. Sport sandals are adequate for some outings (such as the High Line and Jamaica Bay), but for most others they leave much of your foot exposed and vulnerable to poison ivy, thorny plants, rocks, sharp twigs, and malicious rodents.

When it comes to water, err on the side of excess. Hydrate before your hike, carry six ounces of water for every mile you plan to hike, and hydrate after the hike. Pack a couple of small bottles even for short hikes; then you can linger on the trail or take an alternate route and extend your time outdoors.

Although most of these hikes are easy, as the book's title suggests, it doesn't hurt to plan for unpredictable scenarios by carrying, in addition to water, the following items:

Map	Snacks
Band-Aids and ibuprofen	Flashlight (*with extra batteries*)
Pocketknife (*with tweezers, to aid in removing ticks*)	Sunscreen
	Insect repellent

GENERAL TIPS

Whether the point of your outing is to enjoy nature, get some fresh air, or simply exercise, the following tips may enhance your experience:

- Avoid weekends and traditional holidays if possible; otherwise, go early in the morning. Trails that are packed in the summer are often clear during the colder months.

- Before you hit the trail, double-check your map to confirm your bearings.

- If hiking with young children, keep a watchful eye on them at overlooks and by the edge of outcrops.

- Stay on the existing trail.

- Carry your trash out.

- No one is too young for an easy hike. Bear in mind, though, that children do best on flat, short trails. Toddlers who have not quite mastered walking can still tag along, riding on an adult's back in a child carrier. Remember that kids, whatever their age, dehydrate quickly, so make sure you have plenty of fluids for everyone.

- Take your time along the trails, and don't get so caught up in the forest that you forget to see the trees. The suggested hiking time is merely an average; trail conditions, weather, and many other variables may influence the time it takes to complete a trek.

- Never spook animals. An unannounced approach, a sudden movement, or a loud noise will startle most animals, and surprised animals can be dangerous. Remember that you're hiking in their home, so give them plenty of space.

- Keep an eye out for standing dead trees and storm-damaged living trees with loose or broken limbs that can fall at any time.

TRAIL RECOMMENDATIONS

BIRDING HOT SPOTS

01 Central Park North Woods Walk
04 Great Kills Crooke's Point Labyrinth
06 Inwood Hill Park Grand Tour
07 Jamaica Bay West Pond Trail
08 Pelham Bay Islands Loop

11 Teatown Triple
12 Rockefeller Swan Lake Circuit
13 Tallman Hudson River Overlook Trail
16 Cheesequake Natural Area Trail

CHILDREN'S DELIGHT

01 Central Park North Woods Walk
02 Clay Pit Ponds Connector
05 High Line Southern Section
06 Inwood Hill Park Grand Tour
07 Jamaica Bay West Pond Trail
08 Pelham Bay Islands Loop

11 Muttontown Mystery Trail
12 Rockefeller Swan Lake Circuit
13 Tallman Hudson River Overlook Trail
14 Teatown Triple
16 Cheesequake Natural Area Trail
20 Watchung Sierra Sampler

DOGS' PARADISE

01 Central Park North Woods Walk
06 Inwood Hill Park Grand Tour
12 Rockefeller Swan Lake Circuit
14 Teatown Triple

15 Walt Whitman Sampler
16 Cheesequake Natural Area Trail
17 High Mountain Summit Loop
20 Watchung Sierra Sampler

HISTORIC (H) AND RUINS (R) TRAILS

02 Clay Pit Ponds Connector (H)
03 Governors Island History Hike (H) (R)
05 High Line Southern Section (H)
06 Inwood Hill Park Grand Tour (H)
10 Hook Mountain Challenger (H) (R)

11 Muttontown Mystery Trail (R)
12 Rockefeller Swan Lake Circuit (H)
19 Ramapo Lake Ramble (H) (R)
20 Watchung Sierra Sampler (R)

LEAF-PEEPING OPS

01 Central Park North Woods Walk
06 Inwood Hill Park Grand Tour
09 High Tor
12 Rockefeller Swan Lake Circuit

16 Cheesequake Natural Area Trail
17 High Mountain Summit Loop
18 Norvin Green's High Point
19 Ramapo Lake Ramble

ROCK SCRAMBLERS

09 High Tor
10 Hook Mountain Challenger
17 High Mountain Summit Loop

18 Norvin Green's High Point
19 Ramapo Lake Ramble

SCENIC SPECIALS

10 Hook Mountain Challenger
12 Rockefeller Swan Lake Circuit
14 Teatown Triple
16 Cheesequake Natural Area Trail

17 High Mountain Summit Loop
18 Norvin Green's High Point
19 Ramapo Lake Ramble

SOLITUDINOUS HIKES

09 High Tor
10 Hook Mountain Challenger

17 High Mountain Summit Loop
18 Norvin Green's High Point

WATER DESTINATIONS

01 Central Park North Woods Walk
03 Governors Island History Hike
04 Great Kills Crooke's Point Labyrinth
07 Jamaica Bay West Pond Trail
08 Pelham Bay Islands Loop

10 Hook Mountain Challenger
12 Rockefeller Swan Lake Circuit
14 Teatown Triple
16 Cheesequake Natural Area Trail
19 Ramapo Lake Ramble

WILDFLOWERS IN SEASON

05 High Line Southern Section
06 Inwood Hill Park Grand Tour
11 Muttontown Mystery Trail
12 Rockefeller Swan Lake Circuit
14 Teatown Triple

15 Walt Whitman Sampler
18 Norvin Green's High Point
19 Ramapo Lake Ramble
20 Watchung Sierra Sampler

WILDLIFE VIEWING

10 Hook Mountain Challenger
12 Rockefeller Swan Lake Circuit
14 Teatown Triple

16 Cheesequake Natural Area Trail
18 Norvin Green's High Point
19 Ramapo Lake Ramble

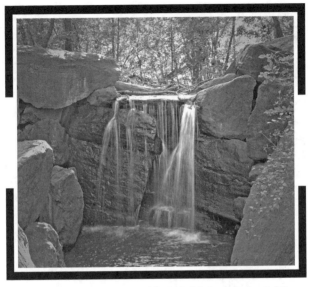

The secluded North Woods section of Central Park features a lovely waterfall.

Manhattan and Proximity

01

Central Park
North Woods Walk

■ OVERVIEW

LENGTH: 1.5 miles

CONFIGURATION: Loop

SCENERY: Old-growth hardwoods, shady streams, a couple of cascades, nonstop beauty

EXPOSURE: Largely shaded

TRAIL SURFACE: Almost completely paved

TRAFFIC: This is *Central Park*—you'll be seeing plenty of people, but far fewer than elsewhere in the park.

HIKING TIME: 2 hours

ACCESS: Open 6 a.m.–1 a.m.; dogs must be on leash no longer than 6 feet and wear license tag and proof of rabies vaccination

MAPS: Posted at Charles Dana Discovery Center and at most major intersections, also at www.centralpark.com/pages/map-it/maps.html

FACILITIES: Restrooms, water fountains, and telephones throughout the park

■ SNAPSHOT

A couple of hours strolling among the rugged rocky outcroppings, picturesque ponds, and musical cascades will transport you to a more tranquil part of the city, and a quieter section of the park. This North Woods tour showcases Central Park's remotest trails, where nature still presides.

■ CLOSEUP

Central Park is so well known, it doesn't really require an introduction. What it really needs is a *reintroduction,* one best undertaken on foot.

With an average of 68,500 people visiting the park every day, you might think that getting away from everyone else would be all but impossible. It is, of course. But in the North Woods section of Central Park, you're such a long way from the park's central attractions that you'll encounter far fewer pedestrians than anywhere else in the domain.

Begin by the Charles Dana Discovery Center (CDDC), at the northern edge of the park, near the 110th Street entrance. On

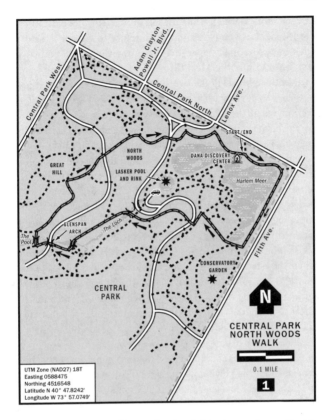

UTM Zone (NAD27) 18T
Easting 0588475
Northing 4516548
Latitude N 40° 47.8242'
Longitude W 73° 57.0749'

exiting the CDDC, walk straight ahead, keeping to the north side of the Harlem Meer. Break right as you near the park's Fifth Avenue entrance, sticking with the shore of the lake. Proceeding south, you will no doubt hear the sounds of traffic along the avenue, just over the wall on your left, while simultaneously enjoying (if it's summer) the abundance of pickerel weed, jewel weed, and many other wildflowers that fringe the water.

On reaching the southern foot of the Meer, roll to the right, still circling the lake. (Straight ahead is a gated access to the

Conservatory Garden, while the left option exits the park.) Proceed straight as you pass a second entrance to the conservatory (this one is normally open), ignoring the right-hand path that continues to hug the Meer. Moving west, away from the water and gently uphill, skip the two spurs to the right that appear just as the wide, paved path crests; then swing left at the third intersection, where the main track comes to an end.

This narrower trail slants southward and uphill and rapidly (in perhaps 40 paces) meets the park road. Cut right and cross the pavement, and in less than ten paces from the far curb your new path forks; go left or right—the two trails will converge in a matter of minutes, as the undulating terrain grows increasingly wild, with bedrock protrusions soaring above the grass, and much of the area appealingly unfenced. (That rock that composes so many of the picturesque outcroppings of the park, incidentally, is Manhattan schist, which was formed 450 million years ago.) Ten steps from where those twin trails rejoin, you should bear right, and in an additional 70 feet spring to the left (more straight than left, actually), rather than going right and recrossing the park road. Still with us? Great, as in a farther 100 feet you should come to a cute little waterfall in a secluded nook, a sweet spot in which to sit awhile and enjoy the dulcet notes of birds bathing in the water.

The trail breaks both left and right, on either side of the cascade, reconnecting higher up the loch. If you swing to the right of the loch, be sure to hang a hard left almost immediately (proceeding straight, or right, carries you through the underpass and into a different area of the park), then continue along the paved walkway for about three minutes to a bridge with a rustic log railing. On crossing the purling stream make a hard right, passing, meanwhile, through an unattractive upheaval of broken and damaged trees, casualties of a freak storm that blew through the park in the summer of 2009. As you amble alongside the now-stagnant stream, the trail draws you through Glenspan Arch, a stone triumph of design created by Calvert Vaux. A double cascade greets you on the other side of that monumental structure, and you can take either the stone steps or asphalt path to get above the falls.

Roll to the right when you reach higher ground, and remain right, breaking away from the foggy green pool that feeds the cascade, rather than following the path that circles it. In five minutes of huffing up the mild but persistent slope, you'll arrive at the aptly named Great Hill, a favorite spot for picnics, ballgames, and sunbathers. Rather than join the throng within the wide track, shift sharply right, heading east-northeast. Turn left at the fork, in about 200 feet, then, after a similar distance, cross the park road and continue straight ahead.

As is the case elsewhere in the park, a number of social trails cut through this area, and you should feel free to explore them. Ultimately, though, you'll want to return to the paved walkway, hike a couple of minutes, then opt for the right fork, to move back toward the road. Hang a right at the fork that overlooks the road, descend the steps, and cross the pavement. That's the Harlem Meer straight ahead, with the back of the CDDC protruding over the water in the distance.

After walking down a second set of stairs, hop left, onto the asphalt path, resuming the circuit around the reed-rimmed lake. Stick with the lakeside trail on reaching the northwest corner of the Meer, maintaining your course toward the CDDC and the conclusion of your hike.

■ TO THE TRAILHEAD

By car: From Central Park's northwestern corner, drive 0.3 miles east on Central Park North/West 110th Street to the Charles Dana Discovery Center on your right. (Street parking may be difficult; for garage parking go to www.bestparking.com.)

By subway: From Grand Central Terminal take the 4 or 5 line to 110th Street.

■ OVERVIEW

LENGTH: 2 miles	**ACCESS:** Year-round, 9 a.m.–5 p.m.; no fees, no bicycles, no pets, no smoking
CONFIGURATION: Double balloon	
SCENERY: Gaping clay-mining pits and ponds, hidden in wetlands and woodlands, surrounded by sandy barrens	**MAPS:** At visitor center; see also nys parks.state.ny.us/parks/attachments/ ClayPitPondsTrailMap.pdf
	FACILITIES: Restrooms, museum
EXPOSURE: Mostly dense canopy but open at Sharrott's Pond	**COMMENTS:** Hikers are not permitted on the horse trails in the preserve, and horses are not allowed on the hiking trails. For further information, call (718) 967-1976, or visit www.nysparks .state.ny.us/parks.
TRAIL SURFACE: Dirt, sand, roots, and wood chips	
TRAFFIC: Generally light	
HIKING TIME: 1 hour	

■ SNAPSHOT

It may be hard to believe, but many of Manhattan's buildings and sidewalks were once made from the clay drawn from the ground of this pocket-size park. The 19th-century brick plant is long gone, replaced now by a fun series of lilting trails that loop by idyllic swamps and peaceful ponds, which serve as a backdrop for a colorful variety of birds and wildflowers.

■ CLOSEUP

One of the most horrific events in New York's past occurred the evening of December 16, 1835, when a fire broke out in a downtown dry goods store. It raged for 15 hours and destroyed nearly 700 buildings, including the post office, the Merchants' Exchange, and most of the financial district.

Enter German immigrant Balthasar Kreischer. As he arrived in the Big Apple following the Great Fire (as it has come to be known), you might say Kreischer made his fortune from a wheelbarrow full of bricks. With wood out of favor, brick (along with iron and stone) became the material of choice for rebuilding the

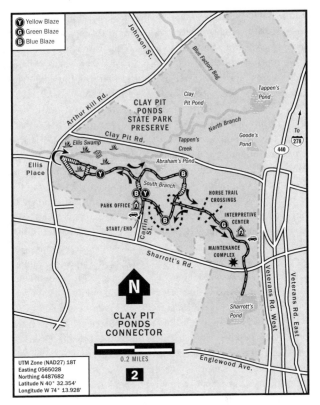

Yellow Blaze
Green Blaze
Blue Blaze

Johnson St.

Blue Factory Bog

Tappen's Pond

CLAY PIT PONDS STATE PARK PRESERVE

Clay Pit Pond

Arthur Kill Rd.

Clay Pit Rd.

North Branch

To 278

Ellis Swamp

Tappen's Creek

Goode's Pond

440

Ellis Place

Abraham's Pond

South Branch

B

HORSE TRAIL CROSSINGS

PARK OFFICE

INTERPRETIVE CENTER

START/END

B

Carlin St.

MAINTENANCE COMPLEX

Sharrott's Rd.

Veterans Rd. West

Veterans Rd. East

N

CLAY PIT PONDS CONNECTOR

Sharrott's Pond

0.2 MILES

2

Englewood Ave.

UTM Zone (NAD27) 18T
Easting 0565028
Northing 4487682
Latitude N 40° 32.354'
Longitude W 74° 13.928'

city, and Kreischer's flame-resistant variety was considered among the best. What, you might ask, does all this have to do with Staten Island's Clay Pit Ponds State Park Preserve? Much of the clay for Kreischer's bricks was mined on this 260-acre property, which was became a state preserve in 1976. You can still see vestiges of clay mining on this short, easy hike, which passes through a delightful mixture of habitats, ranging from wetlands and spring-fed streams to sandy barrens and open fields.

The trailhead is behind the nature center, a shingle- and clapboard-sided house with wisteria growing by its side. Follow the yellow and blue blazes to the left of the picnic pavilion, on the bark-covered path. From initially overlooking a swamp, with a small stream beside you, the trail soon descends through oak, maple, sycamore, briar, birch, beech, and an occasional azalea, to a board-walk where skunk cabbage reigns. Shortly after that, the yellow and blue discs diverge; continue straight, with the yellow ones.

There is a fun lilt to the moss-sided track as it gently rises and falls through this swamp. Bypass the spur to the right—that's where this mini-loop comes to a close—and note the corrugated texture of the land around you, the lingering effects of clay mining. Any squealing of seagulls you may hear overhead is a reminder that the park, on the southwest side of the island, lies very close to the water. The ensuing boardwalk, shaped like an upside-down U, runs 100 feet, passing beneath sweet gum trees, maples, and oaks. Midway along that span is a short spur to the left that leads, in a few paces, to a phragmite-enclosed cluster of swamp ponds; look for frogs and turtles cooling themselves in the water. The main path continues, rising to the right to reconnect with the outbound route. A step or two before that is an appealing nook, to the left, with a bench under pin oaks, in front of a modest cascade.

Persevere along the yellow-blazed trail, swinging left at the close of the loop, and return to where the blue discs earlier branched off. Canter left to cross the 20-foot span, beneath which creeps a slow stream. The track bends abruptly to the right, paralleling that creek; there is a bench and bird-viewing platform on the left, where Abraham's Pond is gradually silting up. If you are lucky, you may observe a muskrat swimming among the cattails and yellow bull-head lilies. Keep to the main path, ignoring both traces on the left. The scrub-filled bowl to the right is one more relic from when this locale was extensively mined for clay.

Three short boardwalks follow, in the dips of the rolling trail, with a pocket meadow succeeding the last one. Walk directly past the bench there, about 100 feet, stopping short of the tree cover opposite; then turn left on the green-blazed trail, an easy-to-miss spur to Sharrott's Pond. Created late in 2002, this out-and-back route is a bit rough around the edges, but the reward for taking it—Sharrott's Pond—is well worth enduring the minor eyesores. The path glides through a pair of livestock barriers in crossing a horse trail, and repeats that same maneuver again in 100 yards; then, in rapid succession, it passes a luminescent field of ferns and a broken-up concrete foundation before meeting a barrier gate. Slip around that, and then swerve right with the meandering trail as it brushes by eastern cottonwoods and some mounds of spent tires and cut-up logs. Continuing right, you stride through another gate and by a park-maintenance building. On pavement now, roll to the right of the brown-sided house dead ahead, hop over the pipe gate, and cross Sharrott's Road.

Less than a minute of walking on the gravel access lane delivers you to an open lawn-like field, with Sharrott's Pond just beyond. Look for great lobelia around the banks of the water, and various types of bladderwort. You may also see an eastern mud turtle, which supposedly is found nowhere else on Staten Island; herons, snowy egrets, and ring-necked ducks frequent this attractive pond, too. Backtrack to the pocket meadow where you jumped off the blue-blazed track, lunging left on it. In about 100 feet, the trail jogs right, past a gate, and descends a touch over erosion-control steps. With a sharp arc to the right, it emerges abruptly by a kiosk at the parking area.

■ TO THE TRAILHEAD

Follow I-278 over the Verrazano Bridge, after which it becomes the Staten Island Expressway, and continue west 6 miles to the junction with NY 440. Drive south on NY 440 about 5 miles to Exit 3 (Bloomingdale Road). Turn left on Bloomingdale, then make a right on Sharrott's Road and another right on Carlin Street. Proceed straight to the park entrance and parking lot, 0.1 mile ahead.

03 Governors Island History Hike

■ OVERVIEW

LENGTH: 2.3 miles	**HIKING TIME:** 1.5 hours
CONFIGURATION: Loop	**ACCESS:** Summer only, from the end of May to mid-October—for latest schedule check www.nps.gov/gois, or call (212) 825-3045
SCENERY: Historic fort; large, grassy expanse; New York Harbor; Buttermilk Channel; Statue of Liberty	
EXPOSURE: Open to sunshine most of the way	**MAPS:** National Park Service maps available in Building 140; also posted at the main kiosk
TRAIL SURFACE: Asphalt	**FACILITIES:** Restrooms in Buildings 140 and 148, adjacent to ferry dock; vending machines in Building 148
TRAFFIC: Hugely popular in good weather, especially on weekends	

■ SNAPSHOT

A historic fort, unparalleled vistas of lower Manhattan and the Statue of Liberty, and plenty of nautical scenery combine to make this a one-of-a-kind stroll. An even more compelling reason to go, however, is the likelihood that a large swath of the island will eventually be developed, filling in a landscape that is, for now, wonderfully open, green, and expansive.

■ CLOSEUP

It may seem inappropriate to describe as a "work in progress" a landmass that served as a military redoubt for nearly 200 years and for an additional 30 after that as a Coast Guard command center. Yet for much of that time, Governors Island has been largely invisible to most New Yorkers. That owes partly to the fact that for many years the island was off-limits, and mapmakers omitted it from their charts of the region. Yet some argue that because Dutch settlers made their way north to Manhattan after first coming ashore at Noten Eylant (as it was first called, on account of the abundance of nut trees), modest little Governors Island gave birth to New York State.

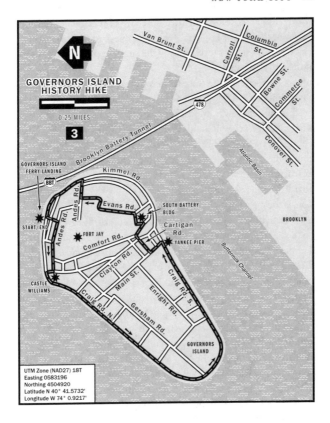

There were about 120 buildings on the island when the Coast Guard finally vacated it in 1997, and much of the fort still stands, incorporated into a 22-acre national monument created in 2001. As for the island's remaining 150 acres, they were sold back to New York in 2003 for the princely sum of one dollar, setting in motion as many development plans as there are colors in a rainbow. One idea that appears to be gaining traction calls for shifting landfill (from buildings soon to be demolished) to convert the currently-flat southern part of the island into a series of interconnected hills, groves, wetlands, and gardens. Before any of that gets under way, however, it is possible—and even advisable—to tour the car-free island on foot or by bicycle during the summer months, beginning at the end of May.

On disembarking from the ferry, strut directly to the left and enter Building 140 to obtain a map of the historic fort area. Then head uphill and away from the wharf to the flagpole and kiosk, where a ferry schedule and a larger map of the entire island are posted. Hang a right there, onto Andes Road. The long building on your right, 110, was constructed as a warehouse to hold munitions for distribution to various military posts along the Atlantic seaboard. The current plan, likely completed by this book's publication, is for it to be converted into artist studios.

Marching onward, you pass three Georgian Revival buildings on the right, formerly officers' and nurses' quarters built in the 1930s. The next structure, the massive brownstone with a rounded façade at the end of the road, is the far more imposing Castle Williams. Similar in appearance to Castle Clinton in Battery Park, Castle Williams was built at the same time, between 1807 and 1811, as part of a network of forts designed to protect New York's harbor.

Saunter to the left on reaching the seawall, but not before taking in the fabulous view of lower Manhattan and, as you circle Castle Williams counterclockwise, the Statue of Liberty. You're now gamboling along North Craig Street, shuffling toward the southern tip of the island, on a wide, paved walkway. Stick with it for the next 20 minutes or so while enjoying an unimpeded vista of Ellis Island, Lady Liberty, and sundry ships cruising up and down the river.

Keep walking alongside the green chain-link fence, ignoring the successive lefts onto Clayton Road and the cutoff to Yankee Pier. Once you have passed the brick apartment houses, most of which are slated for demolition, the view inland opens up, with lush, grassy fields replacing derelict buildings. You may wonder as you meander along what happened to all of the nut trees the Dutch found when they first landed nearly 300 years ago. They were razed by the U.S. military, along with all the other indigenous trees and plants, to allow their cannons a clear range of the surrounding water.

It was only when the fort ceased to be of military importance, in the 1870s, that the ornamental shrubs and trees—a few yews here, sycamores there—were planted. The appearance of benches, red Adirondack chairs and like-colored picnic tables, and hammocks signals your imminent arrival at Picnic Point.

Go ahead, grab a seat and enjoy your lunch. Or, if you failed to pack a picnic, you may be able to find some form of refreshment at one of the nearby concession stands. There's also a great visual feast all around you, not just in the people-watching across the expansive lawn, but also in the sundry water-based sights, from the Statue of Liberty (still!) to the west and Staten Island and the Verrazano Narrows Bridge to your south, to the many boats flitting about the bay. And that's Brooklyn coming into view, over Buttermilk Channel, as you round the point.

The circuit persists along the island's perimeter, with the seawall fence still on the right. When you come abreast of Yankee Pier, near Building 109, scuttle to the left, in the direction of Colonels' Row. The ground beneath you was actually the south shore of the island until the early 1900s, when landfill (dirt and rocks, essentially) from the construction of the Lexington Avenue subway line increased Governors Island to 172 acres from its original 68.

Turn right on Cartigan Street, between Buildings 330 and 333, now heading toward the parade ground. The street ends in front of a buoy, one of the post's most prominent landmarks, with Our Lady Star of the Sea Chapel, a Catholic church, immediately to your right. Bear to the left of the church (a.k.a. Building 309), along the southeast corner of the parade ground; then, in 70 feet, swing left on Barry Road, the first paved option branching off this blacktop.

From the east side of the parade ground, you next stroll by the South Battery (Building 298). Beyond that, dead ahead, is the Chapel of St. Cornelius the Centurion, an English Gothic–style Episcopal church that was dedicated in 1906. Pivot left there, following the pavement to pass behind a series of yellow clapboard-sided houses, officers' quarters that are among the oldest residences on the island. Take the brick walkway at the end of this oak-, maple-, and hemlock-shaded lane, shifting right along the west side of Building 20.

When you reach Nolan Park, where spruce trees, hostas, and black-eyed Susans contribute to the suburban setting, lunge left, now hastening toward Building 105. That grandiose, neoclassical structure across the green is the Commanding Officer's Quarters, and to its left is the Governor's House. A hard left at the end of the blacktop would bring you to Fort Jay; begun as an earthen fort in 1776, it's the island's oldest building. The continuation of the loop, however, lies to the right.

Once by Building 104, you hit the north side of the island (close to Pier 101) in a matter of seconds; turn left. In quick succession you will encounter the octagonal power station (to the right, out on the water), a pedicab stand, a former Coast Guard building, the bike-rental station, and, closing the circuit, the National Park Service visitor center. Wait here for the ferry to return to Manhattan.

■ TO THE TRAILHEAD

By car: To reach lower Manhattan from the East Side, follow FDR Drive south and take Exit 1, Battery Park/Staten Island Ferry. The passengers-only Governors Island Ferry departs from Slip #7 of the Battery Maritime Building, a large green edifice to the left of the Staten Island Ferry terminal. The ferry ride, which is free during the open season (Memorial Day through October), takes ten minutes. (Street parking is scarce; for garage parking go to www .bestparking.com.)

By subway: From Grand Central Terminal take the 4 or 5 line to Bowling Green.

■ OVERVIEW

LENGTH: 2 miles	**HIKING TIME:** 1 hour
CONFIGURATION: Balloon	**ACCESS:** Year-round, dawn–dusk
SCENERY: Thickly wooded labyrinth, sandy beaches, and bay and harbor views	**MAPS:** At ranger station
	FACILITIES: Restrooms, water, and public phone at ranger station
EXPOSURE: Largely open	
TRAIL SURFACE: Sand and dirt	**COMMENTS:** For further information, call (718) 354-4606, or visit www.nps.gov/gate.
TRAFFIC: Light during week; very crowded on weekends	

■ SNAPSHOT

Calling all sun worshippers! You needn't head to the beach, not while the trails of this expansive park are so gloriously sun-struck. The Crooke's Point circuit leads from one shore area to another, with an agreeable overgrowth of vegetation lending a labyrinthine feel to the jaunt. A sensational range of birds twitters and clucks from within the trees, adding to the appeal of this fun, easy walk.

■ CLOSEUP

Great Kills Park is not the place to go if you have a hankering to mosey meditatively deep in the wilds. With hordes of people flocking there, you are hardly likely to find yourself alone on either of Great Kills' two easy, level hiking trails—though they do draw fewer feet than much of the rest of Staten Island's most popular park.

Amateur ornithologists in particular will delight in the wonderful variety of birds that either nest or stop over here, with the Blue Dot Trail, an out-and-back hike that parallels Hylan Boulevard behind a curtain of trees, an especially active birding area. You can pick up its trailhead just west of the entrance parking lot. Then there is Crooke's Point Labyrinth Trail, a nucleus of three paths

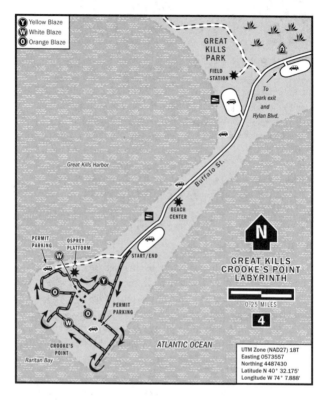

that converge at the center of a scrub-covered spur of land, which juts out into Raritan Bay. Though this small network resembles a labyrinth, you're unlikely to get lost.

The start of the Crooke's Point hike is in parking area G. Facing Nickol's Marina to the west, turn left and walk along the dirt-and-gravel access road. In six or seven minutes, a yellow-blazed path appears on the right, well collared by coastal scrub. Stay with the park road, and when you arrive at the spacious fishermen's parking lot in 100 feet, swing left on the sandy spur to the beach. As you travel toward the shore, check out the two fields that flank you for cowbirds, brown thrashers, and other birds nestling among the bayberry, yucca, and sumac. With the aid of binoculars, Sandy Hook, to the southeast, should be visible from the beach on a clear day. Roll to the right when you reach the open shoreline, and in 40 yards—at the second break in the dunes—cut back to the right toward the parking area. Proceed directly across the lot to the brown post with a white blaze, and enter the trail behind it.

Pitch pine, black birch, black cherry, and flowering fruit trees are tightly interwoven along this shady corridor, contributing a bit of shade and a great deal of natural beauty to the setting. The left fork, arising in a few minutes, leads to the southwestern edge of Great Kills, with nothing but water beyond. Farther along the White Trail, you may have to do the limbo under a few low-hanging branches or outstretched vines before reaching a T. Veer left, now following orange blazes, and after three or four minutes of striding through a tangle of chokeberry, poison ivy, white birch saplings, and—once in a while—yucca, you emerge at the west end of the peninsula. With a marina directly across the bay, head down the sandy trail toward the water, bearing right at the end of the parallel fences that protect the dune grass. Keep to the right, through the small parking lot, and turn right again when you come to the far end of the yellow-blazed route you saw earlier.

Like the other two trails, this track has a secluded, intimate feel, due in large measure to the thriving, jungle-like undergrowth that constantly seems to be offering thorny embraces to passing hikers. A couple of minutes after it drifts under an osprey-nesting platform, the path meets another trail. Stay to the left, with the yellow blazes, and in two more minutes the trail returns you to the dirt-and-gravel access road. Go left and return to parking area G.

■ TO THE TRAILHEAD

Follow I-278 over the Verrazano Narrows Bridge where it joins the Staten Island Expressway. Take the Hylan Boulevard exit, and drive south 4.7 miles to the park entrance and Buffalo Street on the left. Turn there and drive straight, past the ranger station on the right, to the beach-center parking on the left, across from the marina.

■ OVERVIEW

LENGTH: 0.5 miles, so far

CONFIGURATION: Linear or out-and-back

SCENERY: Urban cityscape, wildflower gardens, Hudson River views, plenty of people—some of them unclothed

EXPOSURE: Fairly open

TRAIL SURFACE: Paved with a concrete amalgam

TRAFFIC: Immensely crowded most days, but especially on warm weekends

HIKING TIME: Less than an hour

ACCESS: 7 a.m.–10 p.m.; stairs at Gansevoort, 14th, 16th, 18th, and 20th streets; no dogs, skateboards, skates, or scooters

MAPS: Available at www.thehighline.org/about/maps

FACILITIES: Restrooms at the 16th Street entrance; elevators at the 14th Street and 16th Street entrances; for more information, call (212) 500-6035, or visit www.thehighline.org.

■ SNAPSHOT

A trek along the tracks of an abandoned railway may not sound too alluring, but this one is like no other rails-to-trails hike you've done. It follows a retrofitted stretch of elevated freight line that has been abundantly colored with creative plantings, setting a new standard for the urban paradise while yielding a fresh perspective on a familiar cityscape.

■ CLOSEUP

It's hard to imagine that anyone with an interest in hiking or historic preservation hasn't heard about the High Line. Unlike other rails-to-trails projects, such as the Old Croton Aqueduct and the Briarcliff–Peekskill trails, the High Line doesn't stick close to the ground. Rather, as a reclaimed stretch of viaduct, it soars two to three stories above sidewalk level, along tracks that were abandoned in the 1980s.

This elevated-rail system was built in 1934, raising freight trains above streetside congestions while facilitating delivery of

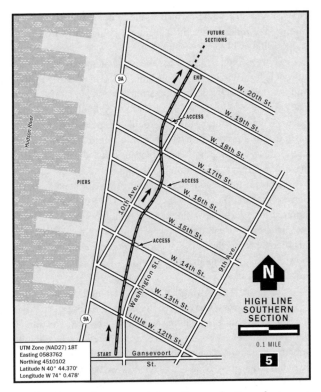

FUTURE
SECTIONS

9A

END

W. 20th St.

ACCESS

W. 19th St.

W. 18th St.

W. 17th St.

ACCESS

W. 16th St.

PIERS

10th Ave.

W. 15th St.

ACCESS

9th Ave.

W. 14th St.

Washington St.

W. 13th St.

9A

Little W. 12th St.

START

Gansevoort
St.

Hudson River

N

HIGH LINE
SOUTHERN
SECTION

0.1 MILE

5

UTM Zone (NAD27) 18T
Easting 0583762
Northing 4510102
Latitude N 40° 44.370'
Longitude W 74° 0.478'

merchandise and raw materials to the production plants scattered around Chelsea and the Meatpacking District. Competi-
tively priced truck transport led shippers to abandon the rail line
in 1980.

The successful drive to save the old elevated rails began in
1999 with the founding of Friends of the High Line, which lobbied
for its preservation as open space. The group gained the support of
City Hall, and by 2005 New York assumed ownership of the property from CSX Transportation, Conrail's successor. The first segment of this projected route, from Gansevoort and Washington
streets to 20th Street, is a mere half mile long. The second section,

from 20th to 30th streets, which is due to open in 2010, will add another half mile. And a third segment, going north from 30th Street, will very likely be worth the wait.

Short as the High Line is, your walk there may well be the most delightful and unusual of any you've had in all of Manhattan. And the slowest. This destination attracts people in numbers normally associated with Times Square at the height of tourist season, and once there, few hurry to leave. You'll understand why once you see it. In part, the attraction has to do with a union of clever design and creative landscaping, which has endowed the space with a sleekly modern, yet oddly apocalyptic appearance.

To begin, join the throng ascending the wide staircase at the Gansevoort Street entrance. Once atop those 46 or so steps, take a moment to absorb the setting around you. Nothing you've read, here or elsewhere, can quite prepare you for the thrilling sight of this altered perspective of the city, and of the apparently anarchic—though actually quite thoughtfully planned—landscaping that covers much of the walk.

From the stairs, swing left, to the dead-end overlook, for a vertigo-inducing view two to three stories above Gansevoort. When you tire of the vista, turn around and proceed north. As you wander along the concrete amalgam–surfaced path, note how the old rails, sometimes mounted on new pilings, artistically overflow with birch trees and sedge grass, coral bells, coneflowers, bee balm, and some 200 other varieties of flowers and plants, as if nature alone were responsible for the plantings. That is, of course, a deliberate illusion, one created by the numerous volunteers responsible for installing and tending the gardens.

Moving north, the first landmark you come to is the Standard Hotel, a trendy hostelry that hovers over the High Line at 13th Street. If the pace slows down here, it's probably because the floor-to-ceiling window exposure of the Standard's rooms has been much publicized, drawing voyeur tourism to this spot. The row of chaise lounges that follows is sometimes referred to as "the beach," and if it's a bright, warm day you'll probably see every chair occupied by sun worshippers.

Just as you reach the next underpass, the High Line separates, the left fork dropping a few steps while simultaneously yielding views of the Hudson River, where an elongated elbow of the track serves as a terrace, complete with tables and chairs. The right fork passes a coffee concession, where organic cupcakes are also available. The forks rejoin a few steps farther, by yet another building underpass.

Keep strolling north, and at 17th Street you'll find one of the High Line's more inventive flourishes: a section of stadium-style seating in a nook to the right. From the tier of benches here, hordes of people stop to socialize or simply stare through the large panes of glass overlooking 10th Avenue, enjoying a view of taxis and other vehicles as if watching a Broadway show. Shuffling along, the meandering route showcases the Empire State Building, which glows gorgeously in late-afternoon light, and—so close you could almost touch it—Frank Gehry's IAC Building.

And then, just like that, you've reached 20th Street and (temporarily) the end of the line, a narrow set of stairs leading down to street level. But if, like so many, you found yourself strangely elevated by your High Line experience, by all means do an about-face and return the way you came, enjoying the High Line life for just a little bit longer.

■ TO THE TRAILHEAD

By car: Follow 9th Avenue south to where Hudson Street forks left. Continue 0.1 mile on Hudson and turn right on Gansevoort Street. After less than 0.2 miles, the staircase to the elevated trail will be on the right. (If street parking is scarce, go to www.bestparking.com.)

By subway: Take the A, C, or E line to 14th Street.

■ O V E R V I E W

LENGTH: 2.3 miles	**TRAFFIC:** Fairly light
CONFIGURATION: Loop	**HIKING TIME:** 1.5 hours
SCENERY: Gigantic trees, rolling terrain, glacially scoured bedrock, plus Hudson River and bridge views	**ACCESS:** Open year-round, no fees
	MAPS: See www.nycgovparks.org/ sub_about/parks_divisions/nrg/ forever_wild/pdf/fw-trailmap-38.pdf
EXPOSURE: Mostly shaded, except for the short path to the Hudson River	**FACILITIES:** Restrooms near main entrance, directly across from the ball fields
TRAIL SURFACE: Macadam much of the way	

■ S N A P S H O T

The dense groves of old-growth poplars, intermingled with a glacially scoured environment, provide a great image of what Manhattan might have looked like before European settlers arrived. Add to that a forest teeming with bird life and wildflowers, plus an undulating terrain that yields stunning views of the Henry Hudson Bridge as well as the Hudson and Harlem rivers, and you've got the makings of a highly memorable hike.

■ C L O S E U P

Inwood Hill Park is one of those urban oases that owe much of their appeal to the fact that few people know of them. That anonymity works in Inwood Hill's favor, for on days when most other Big Apple parks are overrun with all sorts of outdoors enthusiasts, this park offers the opportunity to rub elbows with Mother Nature—while getting away from almost everyone else. Yet this is hardly a pocket park: Inwood Hill covers a whopping 196.4 acres, most of it rather densely forested. Unlike Central Park, Inwood Hill's rolling hills and rocky landscape were never, well, *landscaped*. The sense of wilderness evoked by its dense groves of oaks and tulip trees, its furrowed flanges of protruding bedrock, and its many delicate wildflowers—

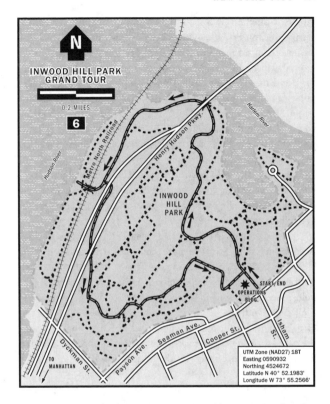

all of that has come about naturally. To be sure, Inwood Hill makes concessions to organized athletics, most notably in the ball fields and tennis courts by its main entrance. But because it's relatively remote, snugly tucked into Manhattan's northern end, the park has long remained invisible to most Gotham residents.

That's surprising, given the rich history of this domain. Eons before the Dutch arrived in the 1600s, local Indians camped in the area; some of their shelters have been found among the rocks in the eastern hills of the park. According to native lore, Inwood Hill is where the Lenape Indians sold Manhattan Island to the Dutch; a plaque commemorating the event is by one of the baseball diamonds. Colonial forces built an earthwork fort near where the Henry Hudson Bridge now touches down within the park, but it fell to British troops during the Revolution and was razed to the ground. Much of the park's land was farmed during the 19th century, and its hills were dotted with country estates and even a library and orphanage. Among the former residents were Ida and Isidor Straus, owners of Macy's, who were on board the *Titanic* and died when it sank. New York acquired the property in 1916, just in time to preserve the island's last surviving salt marsh, where waterfowl cavort during the migratory seasons of spring and fall. As you putter along the network of paved and unpaved trails, keep your eyes open for raccoons, skunks, owls, red-tailed hawks, and—because of a breeding program begun several years ago—maybe even a bald eagle.

Enter the park at Inwood Hill's main entrance, where Seaman Avenue and Isham Street intersect, and walk straight ahead about 100 yards to the flagpole, passing the latrines and basketball courts on your left and the baseball diamonds to the right. On reaching the pole, proceed straight and in less than 60 seconds you will arrive at a junction, with the left fork ascending and the right dropping. Hang a left, noting the many monumentally tall tulip poplars among the oaks and maples. The rocky uplift visible throughout this hike, by the way, was deposited by the Wisconsin Glacier more than 25,000 years ago.

Bear right in about two minutes, just after the paved path levels off, and in less time than it takes to read these words, bear right again. Heading west, the trail forks once more as it brushes up against the base of an impressive rocky bluff. The remnants of Paleolithic shelters were found among those corrugated shelves, as were pottery shards, a few stone artifacts, and the traces of old campfires. Feel free to scramble up there, but when you are finished, hop back on the trail and swing right, following it now to the north.

A few steps beyond the modern-era fire pit, where low concrete columns serve as seats, is the next intersection; climb to the left, ascending the unpaved path that's demarcated by stones (the right returns to the ball fields). This is one of the wilder sections of the park, where wood asters, goldenrod, jewel weed, and Asiatic day lily grow abundantly and poison ivy pretty much reigns. Ignore the many social trails through the understory and go right at the next fork; then, as you near the crest, take a left, the steepest of the three options.

Once atop the hill, head to the right, now back on pavement and on course toward the northwest and the Henry Hudson Bridge. As the path shifts downhill, it passes to the right of the Metropolitan Transit Authority's fenced-in parking area, yielding an impressively up-close view of the bridge. The circuit then swoops east before bending back toward the northwest, where a break in the tree cover yields an awesome panorama of the Harlem River below and the Bronx across the water. Go right at the next junction; then, once you find yourself underneath the erector-set struts of the bridge, keep left (more straight than a hard turn), toward the west and the Hudson River.

Stick with this paved path even as it arcs to the south, providing glimpses as it does so of a couple of train trestles, and then the tracks of the West Side Line, some 60 feet below you, which are used by Amtrak's Empire Connection (among other trains). Pay no attention to the acute left turn by the pair of enormous beech trees at the next junction, proceeding straight instead. In a couple of minutes the path descends to the level of the railroad before gradually climbing again. Continue straight at the next intersection, a kind of triangle, where a left would lead under the southbound lane of Henry Hudson Parkway.

The path brings you to a set of stairs that provides access to a footbridge over the railroad. On descending the staircase on the opposite side, head due west, directly to the sycamore-lined edge of the Hudson River. For proximity to the water, it is hard to do better than this picturesque promenade. Go ahead, grab one of the many benches here and soak up the waterside ambience. When you're ready to resume the hike, retrace your steps to the triangle intersection you passed earlier, and this time venture right, under the parkway and up the stone steps on its far side.

With the narrow path paralleling the highway for the next five or so minutes, any sense of tranquility, or ability to have a conversation, will be hostage to the traffic roaring up and down the twin lanes of the Henry Hudson. Be patient: though this is not the happiest part of the hike, peace will be restored once you sprint under the northbound lane and follow the trail as it gains ground, chugging south, away from the road. Head right at the subsequent slanted T, then turn left in 70 feet.

Now, in what is perhaps the most labyrinthine area of Inwood Hill, the choices come fast and furiously. Worry not, as it doesn't matter that much which way you go, since most trails will eventually bring you back to the ball fields. That said, if you'd like to stick with us to the end, proceed as follows: go straight (or right) rather than left at the next fork, making a left less than a minute after that. Go left again in roughly 70 feet, and in an additional 100 feet make a right; otherwise you'll return to the area of the bridge and highway. Keep right in another 50 feet, finally regaining the main path; walk an additional 30 feet and go right again, at an intersection marked by a whale-size rock. Jog left at the four-way intersection (roughly 65 feet), then left twice more, each turn separated by about 275 feet. Just after you pass a narrow path on the left, where three pylons poke up from the ground, take the right turn, climbing slightly over asphalt. Bear left (the straighter of the two options) at the next spur, and proceed to the stone steps.

Sundry sports fields are visible from here, and on hanging a left at the base of the staircase you will brush by the handball and tennis courts of Emerson Playground. Make a right when you reach the flagpole, in 100 yards, to get back on the path leading to the entrance. The park exit is dead ahead.

■ TO THE TRAILHEAD

By car: Follow US 9/Broadway north to West 207th Street and go left (west) on it. After 0.1 mile make a right on Seaman Avenue. The park's main entrance is 0.1 mile ahead on the left. (Street parking is possible, but for garage parking go to www.bestparking.com.)

By subway: Take the A line to 207th Street.

■ OVERVIEW

LENGTH: 2 miles, including the Terrapin spur

CONFIGURATION: Loop

SCENERY: Views of coastal marshlands and New York City along level, gravel trail flanked by exotic plants and encircling a brackish pond populated with waterfowl

EXPOSURE: Mostly open; some shady trees on the east side in North and South Gardens

TRAIL SURFACE: Packed dirt covered with gravel

TRAFFIC: Very popular on weekends

HIKING TIME: 1 hour (more for serious birders)

ACCESS: Year-round, dawn–dusk; can get breezy in winter; free, but must obtain permit at visitor center; no bikes; no smoking

MAPS: At visitor center

FACILITIES: Restrooms and water at visitor center; water fountain by bird blind near South Garden

COMMENTS: Sunsets can be gorgeous. Bring good binoculars or a spotting scope to watch abundant and fascinating bird life. If you want to hike the East Pond across the road, wear waterproof shoes and go at low tide. For additional information, call (718) 318-4340, or visit www.nps.gov/gate.

■ SNAPSHOT

This hike is for the birds—and for those who love to observe them in all their curious shapes, plumages, and idiosyncrasies. The richest sightings are during spring and fall migrations, when the ponds and surrounding marshlands teem with waterfowl, but this is a refuge of calm worth visiting throughout the year. Exotic plants and colorful wildflowers bloom from spring through early autumn.

■ CLOSEUP

On the surface of a New York area map, it is easy to overlook Jamaica Bay Wildlife Refuge. In spite of its prime position east of Brooklyn and south of Queens, Jamaica Bay's proximity to JFK Airport evokes images of ambling with one's ears stoppered against sonic boom,

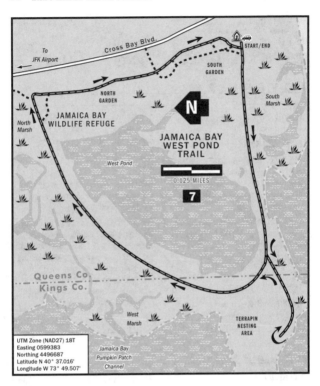

while the sandy soil constantly quakes from crisscrossing jet traffic. Who would willingly walk in such cacophonic conditions?

Well, serious birders, for one. The truth is, flyovers are not as frequent—or nasty—as you might think, and there are many more birds soaring through the air than 747s. The refuge was established in 1951 by the New York City Parks Department, which promptly created two freshwater ponds and transformed what was then barren land into a veritable garden. In 1972, the National Park Service assumed management of the 9,155-acre refuge under the umbrella of the Gateway National Recreation Area, which operates two other units within the metropolitan region. Since then, more than 325 species of birds have been identified in the park.

West Pond is the more accessible of the two principal bird-watching zones, with a 1.8-mile gravel path circling it. Throughout the year, feathered creatures of all stripes, shapes, and colors can be seen by its shore, on its water, and in the surrounding marshlands. But if you are one who knows a booby from a bunting and a grackle from a grosbeak, you should consider timing a visit to coincide with major avian activity. The Park Service notes that evenings in late March are ideal for observing the mating behavior of American woodcocks; a multitude of southbound migrators starts appearing in mid-August; and autumn months are best for seeing songbirds, raptors, and warblers.

Once through with the obligatory registration at the visitor center, pick up the start of the West Pond loop behind the building. Arising immediately are a couple of right-hand turnoffs to the Upland Nature Trail and the South Garden Trail. If you choose to travel counterclockwise, start with the South Garden Trail, which flows in a meandering fashion, first into Upland and then the North Garden Trail before emerging at the northeast corner of the West Pond circuit. A left at that point completes the tour around the pond and marshes. We prefer to roam in a clockwise manner, initially bypassing those two side spurs.

The path is wide and level, with viewpoints spaced between thriving stands of winged sumac and a wondrous array of wildflowers, including the yellowish-orange gaillardia, purple loosestrife, blue vervain, purple gerardia, evening primrose, salt-marsh flea bane, goldenrod, rose mallow, and—perhaps the biggest botanical surprises—prickly pear cactus and flowering yucca. Clearly, this preserve is as much fun for amateur botanists as it is for birders.

Look left toward the South Marsh and you may see such salt-loving waterfowl as snowy and great egrets, yellow-crowned night herons, and possibly an osprey up on the nesting stand, with Gil Hodges Memorial Bridge visible in the distance. In a few dozen yards, the vegetation cloaking the trail opens up, offering greater views of the phragmite-flanked West Pond. The Terrapin Nesting Area spur is farther on to the left (closed during the diamondback terrapin's breeding season—typically midsummer through mid-September); it dead-ends in about 750 feet at an unobstructed view of Manhattan across the bay. As you continue along the loop, the North Garden appears on the right, notable for its invitingly grassy grove of mature willow oaks, cedars, and sweet gum trees.

By all means explore the North Garden trails, since landscaping along the main path becomes less attractive as it parallels the noisy Cross Bay Boulevard back to the parking lot. The North Garden, on the other hand, while offering no further views of the West Pond or saltwater marshes, is a peaceful, less trammeled oasis. Many of its trees (as well as those in the South Garden)—including white birches, cottonwoods, American holly, white pines, and trees of heaven—were planted by the refuge's first supervisor, Herbert Johnson, back in the 1950s and early 1960s.

Now somewhat overgrown, a small warren of trails threads in and out of the thicket, leading, eventually, to a tiny bird pond complete with a viewing blind. This is a fun area of the park to wander around while listening attentively to all sorts of little critters crackling noisily in the underbrush. And since the North Garden, Upland Trail, and South Garden are interconnected, with the West Pond on one side of you and the main path on the other, there's no real chance of getting lost. Just keep moving southward, and soon enough you'll be back by the visitor center.

■ TO THE TRAILHEAD

Exit the Belt Parkway east onto Cross Bay Boulevard (Exit 17) south. Drive 3.6 miles, over the North Channel Bridge, to the signposted refuge entrance and parking lot on the right. Access the trail through the visitor center.

■ OVERVIEW

LENGTH: 2.9 miles	**MAPS:** At Orchard Beach Nature Center during summer
CONFIGURATION: Two loops	
SCENERY: Saltwater marshes, tidal inlets	**FACILITIES:** Several restrooms along Orchard Beach boardwalk, concession stands in summer, picnic areas, tennis courts, golf course, playground, athletic field
EXPOSURE: Mostly shady	
TRAIL SURFACE: Gravel and dirt, boardwalk and grass	
TRAFFIC: On summer weekends, most people remain on Orchard Beach	**COMMENTS:** Bring insect repellent May–September, when mosquitoes reign. For further information, call (718) 430-1890, or visit www.nycgov parks.org.
HIKING TIME: 1.5 hours	
ACCESS: Year-round, dawn-dusk; free admission; Memorial Day weekend–Labor Day $5 parking fee	

■ SNAPSHOT

Giant beech, birch, and tulip trees grace this tranquil oasis with generous shade, which is within a tennis-ball lob of one of the area's more popular beaches and sports complexes. Proximity to a lagoon, the bay, and a salt marsh makes this a birding paradise, especially during the spring and fall migrations, so don't forget to bring your binoculars.

■ CLOSEUP

In the mood for a trivia question? Name the Big Apple's biggest park. *Hint:* it consists of land the city acquired in 1888 and now totals 2,766 acres, including 13 miles of shoreline. If you guessed Pelham Bay Park, you're ready for an appearance on *Jeopardy!*

Of the 28 estates that once lined Pelham Bay, only the Bartow-Pell Mansion (circa 1840) remains. Which is not to suggest that this coastal park is largely undeveloped. On the contrary, visitors with a penchant for play can indulge in a panoply of

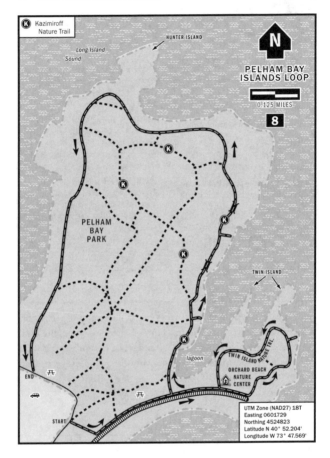

pursuits, including tennis, basketball, golf, beach-bathing, even horseback-riding. Did we overlook hiking? There is that, too, with the excellent Hunter Island and Twin Island double-dip just off Orchard Beach.

Start at the northeast end of the parking lot and stroll toward the water. No, this is not going to be a sandy beach walk; when you hit the concrete boardwalk, turn left and go to the Orchard Beach

Nature Center, at Section 2 of the beach, to pick up an interpretive brochure. Continuing along the boardwalk, hang a left at the next break in the inland side of the railing and take the middle trail, the widest of three options, rapidly entering into the shade of oak, birch, black locust, and shagbark hickory trees, with beggar squirrels scrambling around by your feet. This is Twin Island, which is not actually an island at all. It was—until 1947, when the parks commission filled the water between it and the mainland with rocks, effectively extending the peninsula. (A similar stunt had been pulled on nearby Hunter Island, 13 years earlier.) Nonetheless, the contrast between the calm of this peaceful retreat and the rollicking sounds of the picnic parties and beach-bathers beyond is sharp enough to feed the illusion of being on a distant speck of land.

Ignore the social trails that have been worn into the loamy soil, sticking instead with the main track as it passes a patch of phragmites and wild blackberries before arriving at a spur on the right, which leads to the rocky, glacier-scoured shore. Go ahead and explore this scenic spot, which is attractive despite all the plastic and other flotsam; then return to the path, which soon arcs westward (left), meanwhile skirting additional waterside access points. Within a minute or three, as the trail curves southward, you are delivered onto the sandy beach, with a tidal inlet—look for herons and egrets—to the right. Keep moving south, until you reach the crotch of the inlet, where the path splits in three: take the right fork and, now heading west, rock-hop over the tidal stream. Leap left at the next intersection, by the interpretive sign about shore birds, to join a wide trail, and stay with this as it emerges by the nature center.

The next stage of this convoluted course lies to the right, about 100 yards along the boardwalk. March inland directly opposite the sign for Section 3 of the beach, by another gap in the barrier, and move toward the woods, steering to the right of the picnic area. In a jiffy you'll be under a dense canopy of mature shade trees, on the first leg of Kazimiroff Nature Trail, where numbered posts correspond to descriptions in the brochure you picked up at the nature center. Great white egrets and other waterfowl fish and nest in the weeds and shallows of the surrounding marshes, and with the abundance of spurs to water and marsh viewpoints, bird sightings almost as ubiquitous as the swarms of mosquitoes.

Toward the center of Hunter Island, a tangle of sassafras, beech, and black birch—many aged and goitered—lends an air of seclusion to this part of the park. Feel free to dart inland and explore the rat's maze of interlacing trails; with water on three sides of the peninsula, you'll have to work hard to get lost. For the easiest water access, though, hang around the perimeter, sticking to the right at almost every major junction. Head through the first such intersection, which occurs just as you encounter a cluster of mature tulip trees. Bear right at the next fork, brushing by a massive oak and over a pair of long wooden bridges. At the four-way crossing, continue straight as the path descends perhaps 12 feet over a large, stele-like stone, then bends left, yielding glimpses of a salt marsh and the north end of the bay.

Proceed through the intersection just after a superannuated tulip tree; the left leg returns to the Kazimiroff, while the right trace leads to the water and a picnic table in the sandy marsh. The main trail circles to the left, then parallels the lagoon and begins a great stretch for watching birds and boats—have your binoculars handy. Continue walking southward, by majestic oaks and a few mature cottonwoods, keeping the cord grass and water to your right. The odd popping sound of tennis balls indicates the trail's imminent end by a cluster of white birch trees and picnic tables at the north side of the parking lot.

■ TO THE TRAILHEAD

By car: Take I-95 north to Exit 8B (Orchard Beach/City Island) and follow the signs to Orchard Beach, driving approximately 2.5 miles to the large parking lot on the right. Continue straight across the lot and park by the tennis courts. Orchard Beach lies directly beyond.

By subway: From Grand Central Terminal take the 6 line to its last stop at Pelham Bay.

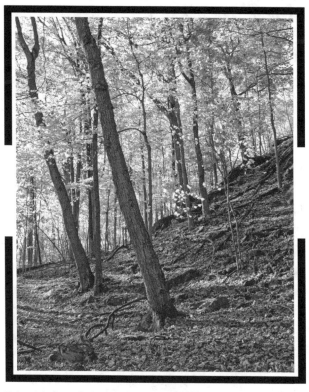

Teatown Lake Reservation is popular for its abundant wildflowers and spectacular fall colors.

Nearby New York

■ OVERVIEW

LENGTH: 2.7 miles	**MAPS:** At park office; USGS Haverstraw
CONFIGURATION: Out-and-back	
SCENERY: Expansive views	**FACILITIES:** Toilets, public phone, and water available by the park's main entrance
EXPOSURE: Mostly dense canopy in summer, sun-struck in winter	
TRAIL SURFACE: Largely rocky	**COMMENTS:** In icy or snowy conditions, the rock scramble descent off the north side of High Tor, leading to Low Tor, may be extremely hazardous. Call (845) 634-8074 or visit www.nys parks.state.ny.us/parks.
TRAFFIC: Fairly light weekdays, heavy weekend visitation	
HIKING TIME: 2.5 hours	
ACCESS: Year-round, dawn–dusk; no fee; foot traffic only; pets must be leashed	

■ SNAPSHOT

While the struggle years ago to prevent the demolition of High Tor inspired a hit Broadway play, it's the views from its peak that are the real showstoppers, with the Hudson River flowing directly below and the Catskills and Shawangunks visible far to the northwest. Especially enjoyable are the scramble up High Tor's summit over wrinkly volcanic basalt, and the deep-woods flavor of its surroundings.

■ CLOSEUP

Like most hikers, we don't relish chewing the same scenery twice, and as a rule we'll opt for a good loop over an out-and-back trek any day. There are exceptions to every rule, however, and a few linear romps—Fitzgerald Falls, Sterling Ridge, and Sandy Hook (see our companion guide, *60 Hikes within 60 Miles: New York City*) come readily to mind—are quite exceptional indeed. The jaunt to High Tor (and Low Tor, if you have the time) belongs in this category of out-and-back hikes that are so memorable, and memorably rewarding, that we simply can't exclude them from this volume.

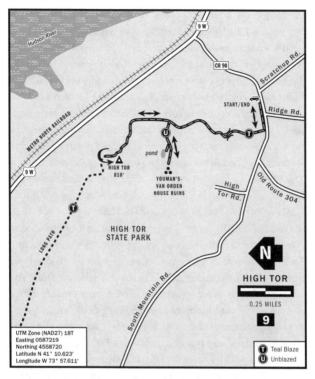

Once out of your automobile, walk west, away from the Hudson River, sticking to the right shoulder of the road. After the fourth telephone pole, the teal blazes of the Long Path (LP) jag to the right, past a large tree and into the forest. The trail, threading among myriad oak, birch, and beech trees, as well as wild violet and garlic mustard, is rocky to start with, as it bumps over duckboard planks and begins to gain elevation. The mild ascent continues through secondary growth, including a smattering of cedars, before leveling off in about ten minutes (after a slight gain of 150 feet) amid a rumpled, corrugated landscape where wild turkeys often roam. An unblazed spur to the left, indicated by a large sign, leads, in less than a quarter mile, to the site of

the Youman's–Van Orden (a protector of High Tor) House and a former winery. Little more than a tiled floor remains, but the adjacent
pond is attractive and lends the short detour some extra value.

Back on the main trail, the uphill slog resumes for another
three to five minutes before you reach the shoulder of High Tor, with
a filtered view of the Hudson straight ahead. The LP then lunges left,
over an intimidating amount of rocky scree accumulated at the peak's
base. The path skirts the worst of that obstacle, looping to the left of
the rocks while giving you an opportunity to observe chipmunks
at play in and around the chinks and crevasses of the moraine heap.
The LP then moves on to another node, then a third, higher one,
before cresting atop High Tor. This loge-level vantage point of the
Shawangunk range to the north, and the Hudson River to the east,
was used by colonial troops as a signal post during the Revolutionary
War to alert people to the comings and goings of the British army.
Today it is favored as a local party spot, to judge by the distressing
amount of graffiti smeared across the volcanic substrate under your
feet. The vultures flying by at eye level are a more thrilling distrac-
tion, as well as the blue azure and mourning cloak butterflies that
show up in warm weather. That rock quarry far below you to the
southeast, by the way, is a stark reminder of what might have happened to this peak if not for the labors of conservationists.

This is the turnaround stage of the hike. (If you'd like to go on
to Low Tor, the trail continues on the north side of the dome, where
the scramble down can be seriously challenging when there's snow
or ice on the path.) To return to your car, simply retrace your steps.

■ TO THE TRAILHEAD

Cross the George Washington Bridge on I-95 south, taking Exit 74,
then merging onto Palisades Interstate Parkway North. Take Exit 4
onto the US 9W north ramp. Go left on US 9W north/Palisades
Boulevard and follow it 14.5 miles to South Mountain Road/CR
90, a sharp left uphill. Drive 0.5 miles, then park on the right shoulder, just before the intersection with CR 23.

10   *Hook Mountain Challenger*

■ OVERVIEW

LENGTH: 5.8 miles	**TRAFFIC:** Very light midweek, but can get crowded on summer weekends
CONFIGURATION: Loop	
SCENERY: Dense hardwood forest, a rock-strewn ridge, an extended stretch by the Hudson River	**HIKING TIME:** 3 hours
	ACCESS: Year-round; dogs must be leashed
EXPOSURE: Well shaded, except for a few open summits; morning sun along the river	**MAPS:** Posted and for sale at park office in parking field 2
TRAIL SURFACE: Packed dirt, granite bedrock, crushed cinder	**FACILITIES:** Restrooms at Nyack Beach State Park, 4 miles into the hike

■ SNAPSHOT

Breathtaking vistas of the Hudson River from a traprock ridge 702 feet up are just one reason to choose this excellent hike. Another is the extended promenade alongside the water on the back half of the loop. Add to that an assortment of plants that might leave a botanist slack-jawed with wonder, and we're willing to bet that after one tour of Hook Mountain, you too will be hooked.

■ CLOSEUP

Hook Mountain, situated along the Hudson River at the lower end of the Palisades, owes its name to the Dutch settlers who dubbed it Verdrietige Hoek ("Sad Corner"), because this perilous stretch of the Hudson claimed many lives. What was sad for the Dutch very nearly became sadder still for the mountain itself. That's because after its historical peak during the Revolutionary War, when the crest served as both a signaling point and a sanctuary for patriots, Hook Mountain became a focus of various development schemes. By the 1830s, for instance, nearby Rockland Lake was the site of a thriving ice industry, and the Knickerbocker Ice Company, with

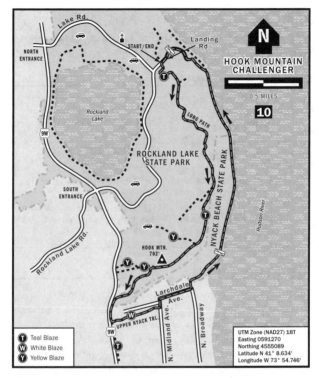

more than 2,000 people on its payroll, used the Hook to run cakes of ice down to the Hudson River to awaiting transport ships. That was just in winter. Summertime placed other pressures on the promontory: brickyards in Haverstraw plumbed the Palisades for clay, leaving behind pockmarked ground and land denuded of trees. In 1846 alone, Hook Mountain and the Tors to the north were stripped of 11,000 cords of wood, fuel used to power the brickyards' furnaces. An even worse threat, however, was posed by the 31 quarries operating in this area of the Hudson that used rock-crushing machinery and dynamite to reduce awe-inspiring monoliths to heaps of gravel. George Perkins, head of the Palisades Parks Commission, spearheaded a grassroots campaign to save the bluffs, convincing wealthy patrons (including the Harriman and Rockefeller families) to donate to the cause. Thanks to his efforts Hook Mountain was saved, and today, after years of augmenting the holdings, the state park totals 676 acres of mostly undeveloped woodland.

On exiting your car, walk to the kiosk on the east side of the parking area and pick up the teal blazes of the Long Path (LP). Follow them to the right, passing a series of concrete foundations as the trail heads south, and plan to remain on the LP for most of the first half of this hike. The 1,243 feet of elevation you gain on this trek (the bulk of it on the LP) begin gradually, with so gentle a slope you may feel as if you're climbing a series of low steps, albeit grass-covered ones. The easy grade of this stretch owes to an overlapping of the LP with some of the old forest roads that once coursed through here. You'll see evidence of those road constructions early on, as you amble past a series of magnificent old retaining walls, in which the remaining stonework is still so solid it could serve as a sidewalk. The tranquility and relative solitude of this setting are in striking contrast to that time, more than a century ago, when the hill was bereft of trees and 3,000 men traversed the lanes, hollering greetings to each other as they hauled wood and clay, or transported ice.

The views of the Hudson River are rather limited when you reach what seems to be the crest of the ridge, given that the LP lies in a grooved track, with higher ground (basaltic diabase, actually) on either side of it. Keep plugging onward, and as the forest road makes a hairpin turn to the left, stick with the teal blazes of the narrower path to its right. Within a minute of scaling this, the steepest section of the trail thus far, you will be on the true spine of the ridge. Stick with the LP as it arcs to the right, southbound, then bear left on the spur, ten paces ahead. This short conduit leads to a rocky shelf of an overlook, where you can enjoy your first unobstructed vista of the river.

More—and better—panoramas await farther down the LP. The ridge peaks at a fine formation of basaltic traprock, a grass-fringed, sun-exposed spot that towers 702 feet above the Hudson. The next viewpoint, while lower, is even more stunning and offers glimpses, from its basaltic terrace, of both the river and an extended patch of shoreside real estate, including much of Upper Nyack to the south. Because of the sheer drop of several hundred feet, by the way, you'll want to keep a keen eye on any little ones who may have accompanied you to this point. The same holds true of the ensuing stretch as it drops down over a ragged, rock-filled bit of trail. Once you're by the worst of that debris, the path forks, with a yellow-blazed route edging to the right. Unless you'd like to bail out back to Rockland State Park, bear left, sticking with the teal tags.

From this dip the LP resumes its uphill surge, continuing to adhere to the Palisades' ridgeline. Though the trail is much over-grown here in summer by vines and various weeds, you may spy such plants as asters, yarrow, butter-and-eggs—even yucca. Prickly pear cacti grace the next peak, a visual reinforcement of how hot this sun-struck spot can get in the warmer months. There's another fork just below this crest, once you're past a scree-filled patch. Keep left, on the LP, and in a few minutes the trail levels off and merges with another forest road.

Look for the three white blazes of the Upper Nyack Trail on a tree to the left, just as the path narrows to single-file. Turn there, finally departing the LP. After snaking downhill among black birches, the Upper Nyack enters an undeveloped berm of trees, a linear swamp hemmed in by a residential neighborhood on one side, a paved road on the other. (Look for the periwinkle-blue flowers of lobelia in summer.) Once you cross a couple of duckboards, the trail spits you out on North Midland Avenue. Look to the left for a white blaze painted on the back of a street sign and head that way.

Continue straight on this paved road, bypassing the first left (which leads to a housing development), until you reach the stop sign by a dark-brown log cabin, one of several buildings within the domain of Marydell Faith and Life Center, a Christian retreat and conference facility. Swing right here on Larchdale Road and stick with it all the way to the next stop sign, where the white blazes (painted on telephone poles) direct you to the left. The Hudson River should now be on your right, while the Palisades tower impressively, imposingly, directly ahead and above.

The white blazes end in about 250 feet, at the entrance to Nyack Beach State Park. Veer sharply right at the gatehouse, heading toward the beach. You'll encounter some picnic tables as you draw closer to the water, and a stairway leading to the shore across from the stone office building. The park road ends by an enormous structure (last chance to use the restrooms!), even as the pavement continues to flank the Hudson's western shore. Mosey ahead on what is now a multiuse walkway, the asphalt eventually devolving to cinder, in much the way the sycamores that line the promenade yield to sumac and other scrub. Note the massive boulders and heaps of talus to your left: some of this debris has fallen from the towering bluff, and much was left behind when the quarries closed.

Eventually, after the trail rambles about 1.25 miles along the riverfront, patches of pavement resurface just as the path begins a gradual ascent. Ignore the two successive spurs to the left when the path levels off; then go left at the third junction (about 35 paces from the second spur), remaining with the main track. (The right option at this wishbone fork descends toward the Hudson and leads to the Haverstraw Trail in 3.5 miles.)

Stick with the road as it doglegs around a brownstone building, disregarding the unpaved track on the left, and meander with it, eventually gaining modest elevation. Four minutes after you put the brownstone residence behind you, the parking area should come into view.

■ TO THE TRAILHEAD

Cross the George Washington Bridge on I-95 south, take Exit 74, and merge onto Palisades Interstate Parkway North. Then take Exit 4 onto the US 9W north ramp. Go left on US 9W north (Palisades Boulevard) and follow it 11.3 miles to the park entrance on the right. After entering, veer left and follow Rockland Lake Road 1 mile, past the park office and Parking Field 2, to Landing Road. Turn left, drive 0.1 mile, and park on the right side.

■ OVERVIEW

LENGTH: 3.3 miles

CONFIGURATION: Double loop

SCENERY: Mysterious ruins and six different habitats, including wet woodlands, rolling fields, kettle ponds, and upland forests

EXPOSURE: Sheltered at the start, then exposed in fields, followed by more tree cover

TRAIL SURFACE: Grass, roots, sand, pebbles, and plenty of mud in spring

TRAFFIC: Light-moderate, except when school groups are exploring grounds

HIKING TIME: 1.5 hours

ACCESS: Year-round, 9 a.m.–4:30 p.m.; no fee; no pets; no bicycles

MAPS: At nature center

FACILITIES: Restrooms and water behind nature center

COMMENTS: Bridle paths and cross-country-skiing trails wind through the preserve. For further information, call (516) 571-8500, or visit www.nassaucountyny.gov/Parks/WhereToGo/preserves/north_shore_preserve/Muttontown_Pres.html.

■ SNAPSHOT

You don't have to be a fan of obscure Albanian history to enjoy wandering the woods of Muttontown, not with such an appealing variety of habitats tucked into the domain. A vast network of trails and old estate lanes weaves through swampy swales, miniature savannas, a rhododendron jungle, some glacial deposits, and even a few ghostly ruins. Of course, if you do have a thing for unsolved mysteries, so much the better.

■ CLOSEUP

Thumb through the brochures at Muttontown's nature center, and you will learn that the 550-acre preserve runs the gamut of habitats, from open fields and lowland swamps to rolling hills, kettle ponds, and upland forests. One pamphlet talks about the variety of animals in Muttontown; another boasts of the birds that nest there. There is even a brief account of how the preserve came into being. What you won't find is any mention of the ruins of Knollwood, the

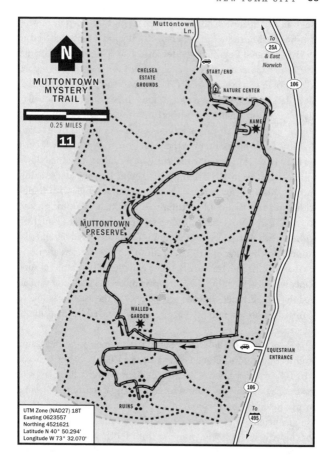

international intrigue surrounding King Zog, rumors of hidden treasure, and an unsolved murder.

To call Knollwood an estate would be to injure it through understatement. Built in 1907 by Charles Hudson, a venture capitalist, Knollwood was a 60-room granite palace that combined such myriad architectural flourishes as Italian Renaissance, Greek

Revival, and Spanish Churrigueresque. Lying at the center of what is now the Muttontown Preserve, Knollwood was purchased in 1951 by Ahmed Bey Zogu, better known as King Zog of Albania. Zog, who had a penchant for poker and perfumed cigarettes (reportedly smoking an average of 150 a day), became president of Albania in 1925 and proclaimed himself king three years later. Not all of his subjects were delighted by this turn of events, so to consolidate power, Zog put each of his four sisters in command of an army division, while his mother ran the royal kitchen—just to make sure his food wasn't tampered with. Still, Zog was almost gunned down by two assassins in 1931, and by 1939, after Italy invaded Albania and defeated its army in two days, he "retired" to England, bringing with him a fair balance of his country's bullion. It was during a visit to the US in 1951 that King Zog saw Knollwood and bought it with—so it was rumored at the time—"a bucket of rubies and diamonds," to the tune of $102,800. Although Zog reportedly never lived at Knollwood, treasure hunters, convinced that more of such booty was hidden within the domain, climbed the walls and vandalized the establishment beyond repair. In 1955 the estate was sold to Lansdell Christie, a mining tycoon, who later razed the mansion to the ground.

More recently, in November 2001, six men were practicing orienteering in Muttontown when one saw a glint of bone beneath a tree—part of a human skeleton hidden below a light layer of leaves. The authorities were summoned, and determined that the corpse belonged to a woman of approximately 35 years, 5′1″ to 5′3″ in height. The victim—she had been murdered, the police concluded—was missing an upper front tooth, in addition to the metal or plastic denture that would have filled the gap. With few clues to go on, the case remains open.

You won't require a deerstalker cap and a pal named Watson to follow the scent in this beautiful sanctuary—sturdy-soled walking shoes and a park map should suffice. Grab a map off the rack on the back porch of the nature center abutting the parking area; then turn around and face the woods. The trail to the right is the shorter interpretive path; to the left is the larger part of the park.

The track bends to the left, initially following the contours of a chain-link fence. Bear left shortly at the wide fork, then roll right at the next junction, exchanging the dirt for a grassy path. Ignore the trace to the right as you cruise through a cluster of birch trees, maples, cedars, and pines on the way to a T. Hang a right there, then a hard right again in a dozen steps, when you reach the boundary fence. On swinging left at the ensuing intersection, in 200 yards you will find yourself in an area of flowering dogwoods, oaks, and an occasional fruit tree. Steer right at the fork, marked by a rare trail blaze, and after striding 150 feet go right at the subsequent fork, now moving toward an open field. Keep left at the next junction, continuing along the west side of the meadow, and proceed through the intersection about 30 yards ahead.

Remain with this open stretch for several minutes, eventually passing a couple of horse corrals. Turn right, directly after the kiosk by the equestrian parking area, onto the broad dirt lane, and bypass the spur to the right that appears almost immediately. The easy walking along this maple-shaded carriage road lasts several minutes, until the trail begins to bend toward the north, whereupon you'll turn left onto a narrower path. This route enters a labyrinth of trails where much of the fun derives from exploring off the beaten track. Saunter left at the four-way intersection, and after a couple of minutes make a right at the fork. From hiking on an overgrown estate road lined with aged apple trees, you are now treading on a narrower track fringed by rhododendrons and ivy. The forest grows wilder as you break to the right at the next fork, with yews dwarfed by a handful of cyclopean pines and beech trees.

And then—suddenly—you are standing among the ruins of Knollwood, with two raised columnar temples flanking a low stairway. Stroll south of the stairs to the overgrown bunker, then retrace your steps and head north between the two temples, while trying to imagine what this looked like more than half a century ago when it was lavishly landscaped with reflecting pools and formal gardens, marble fountains, Greco-Roman statues, and ivy-filled urns. Stick with the trace that extends north above the stairs; it leads to an imposing wall. A baroque gargoyle fountain leers from its center, with symmetrical staircases—now collapsed—rising on either side. This is all that remains of the mansion itself. The trail resumes to the left as you face this crumbling edifice, swooping around its far side. Dart left at the T with the asphalt-covered lane, and reenter the rhododendron forest. Stay with this until the four-way intersection (you met this same crossing from the opposite direction on the way to the ruins), where you venture left and, in 75 feet, left again at the T. Take the middle of three choices at the upcoming junction; it brings you to the front of what is listed on the map as a walled garden, yet another remnant of the Knollwood era.

To continue, cut left of the garden wall; when the trail breaks toward the west, bear right, walking north. Then take the second option to the left (avoiding the open expanse), go left at the post, and make yet another left (once more skirting the field). As you near a chain-link fence, go right. Bypass the subsequent right and instead hang a left at the meadow. Once through that, turn left at the T and left again at the fork that follows. Take the moderately steep spur to the right a minute or two later; this side trip ends atop a kame (glacial deposit), at an elevation of 220 feet. Return to the main track and jag left at the next fork; you are now on familiar turf, backtracking along the first leg of the hike.

■ TO THE TRAILHEAD

Follow the Long Island Expressway (I-495) east to Exit 41 and NY 106 north. Continue on NY 106, driving 4.1 miles to the intersection with NY 25A (Northern Boulevard). Go left, and after 0.1 mile turn left again onto Muttontown Lane. Drive 0.2 miles—through two stop signs—to the preserve entrance on the right. Veer left at the fork into the parking area.

12 Rockefeller Swan Lake Circuit

■ OVERVIEW

LENGTH: 2.2 miles	**ACCESS:** Year-round, 8 a.m.–dusk; $5 parking fee or Empire Passport; no bicycles; pets must be leashed
CONFIGURATION: Balloon	
SCENERY: Carriage roads showcase a lake, deciduous forests, and open fields	**MAPS:** At visitor center and on www.friendsrock.org; USGS White Plains
EXPOSURE: Mostly shady	**FACILITIES:** Restrooms, water, and public phone at visitor center
TRAIL SURFACE: Gravel and cinder	**COMMENTS:** For further information, call (914) 631-1470 or visit www.nysparks.state.ny.us/parks.
TRAFFIC: Crowded on weekends	
HIKING TIME: 1 hour	

■ SNAPSHOT

This walk travels over wide, smooth carriage lanes, but don't be fooled. Rockefeller's scenery runs the gamut, from a glimmering jewel of a lake to the backwoods beauty of rock-studded beech forests and lush meadows. With many, many miles of trails, this is a great spot for short strolls or all-day outings.

■ CLOSEUP

The distance between Rockefeller Center and Rockefeller State Park is only 23 miles. It might as well be 23 *light years,* though, for all the similarity they bear to each other. The immensely popular 1,000-acre park boasts a broad mix of habitats, including woodlands, wetlands, grassy meadows, and a 24-acre lake, with hikers rubbing elbows with joggers and equestrians on its 20 miles of carriage lanes. As for Rockefeller Center, well, you already know about that.

The preserve was originally part of the Rockefeller family's Pocantico Hills estate before being deeded to New York in 1983. Almost all the trails are graded carriage lanes, and thus rugged hiking boots won't be necessary. That said, this is one dazzling domain,

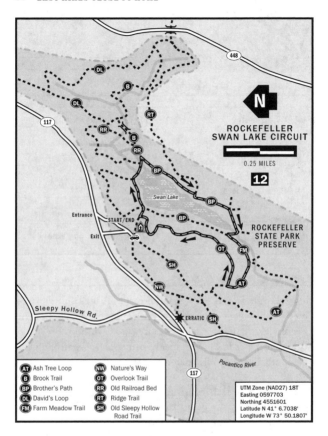

ROCKEFELLER
SWAN LAKE CIRCUIT

0.25 MILES

12

ROCKEFELLER
STATE PARK
PRESERVE

Swan Lake

Entrance

START/END

Exit

Sleepy Hollow Rd.

ERRATIC

Pocantico River

AT Ash Tree Loop		**NW** Nature's Way	
B Brook Trail		**OT** Overlook Trail	
BP Brother's Path		**RR** Old Railroad Bed	
DL David's Loop		**RT** Ridge Trail	
FM Farm Meadow Trail		**SH** Old Sleepy Hollow Road Trail	

UTM Zone (NAD27) 18T
Easting 0597703
Northing 4551601
Latitude N 41° 6.7038'
Longitude W 73° 50.1807'

laced with more than enough loops to let you enjoy a workout of
whatever length you choose.

Stop by the visitor center to pick up a map. The trails are
(mostly) well signposted, but a map is advisable to get the most
out of this 2.2-mile jaunt. Continue past the kiosk to the pastoral
Swan Lake, where lilies dot the water and oaks and goldenrod
thrive by its cattail-lined shore. Follow the left side of the lake, on
Brother's Path, and just after crossing its grass-covered dam make
a right, still hangin' with the Bro as you circle the lake clockwise.

The well-groomed look of the lake area, with the lawn snipped just so, gradually gives way to a wilder forestland appearance the farther you go, as smartweed, jewel weed, various wildflowers, ferns, and sassafras begin to pop up in the understory.

Ignore the Ridge Trail, on the left, sticking with the lakeside Brother's Path for now. At the next intersection, a four-way junction, swing right, continuing to adhere to the Brother's route. Do the same again in another 100 yards, loping toward the southern end of the lake, which is, for the moment, obscured from view. Then, in 50 additional yards, break to the left, away from the water, onto Farm Meadow Trail, a straight, wide track with a stream (run-off from the lake) coursing by on your left.

Turn right onto Ash Tree Loop at the four-way intersection, in another three to four minutes, as Farm Meadow proceeds straight and an unblazed trail branches to the left. Here begins the first sustained climb of the hike, though the elevation gain is nominal. From an open field to your right, the somewhat narrow path passes among an array of oaks, fruit trees, sumac, and wild grapes before meeting the Overlook Trail, where you jog to the right. The uphill slog continues, albeit gradually, as the Overlook Trail draws by a low concrete bunker, a cistern that was built years ago as an emergency water supply for nearby Sleepy Hollow. On putting that behind you, keep an eye out for deer, birds (bluebirds like to nest in the houses posted here), and wildflowers (butter-and-eggs, in particular, thrive from mid- to late summer).

From squiggling indecisively toward the north-northwest, the path finally asserts itself in a grand swoop to the northeast, moving back toward Swan Lake. On reaching the kiosk, near the lakeside, veer left, retracing your earlier steps to the parking area.

■ TO THE TRAILHEAD

Follow I-87 north and take Exit 9 for Tarrytown. Turn left on NY 119, heading west. After 0.25 miles, go right on US 9 north and drive 3.5 miles, then veer right onto NY 117, just after Phelps Hospital. The park entrance is 1 mile farther, on the right.

OVERVIEW

LENGTH: 2.3 miles

CONFIGURATION: Elongated balloon

SCENERY: Dense deciduous forest growing on rocky slopes overlooking the west bank of the Hudson River and Piermont Marsh grasslands

EXPOSURE: Tree cover all the way

TRAIL SURFACE: Dirt, rocks, roots in the first half, level cinder on return

TRAFFIC: Heavy on summer weekends

HIKING TIME: 1 hour

ACCESS: Year-round, 8 a.m.–dusk; third weekend in June–Labor Day, $5 per car; pets must be muzzled and leashed

MAPS: At gatehouse and office; New York–New Jersey Trail Conference, Hudson Palisades Trails

FACILITIES: None along trail, but restrooms in picnic areas and athletic field are open April–November; vending machines in summer; playground, basketball court, pool, track

SPECIAL COMMENTS: The riverside part of this trail overlaps the Long Path, a 350-mile-long (and growing) trail that starts at the George Washington Bridge and leads to the Mohawk Valley, near Albany.

SNAPSHOT

Stellar views and prime, private picnic spots don't come any easier than this level walk to a high overlook of the Hudson River. Birding and boat-watching are extra attractions, as is the possibility of an extended campaign along a piece of the Long Path, which intersects the trail.

CLOSEUP

We've all heard the argument at one time or another. It starts with a rhetorical question; something on the order of, what's the dividing line between a hike and merely a walk? Some people are guided by distance, others by the degree of effort involved. As far as we're concerned, that's like trying to determine which came first, the chicken or the egg.

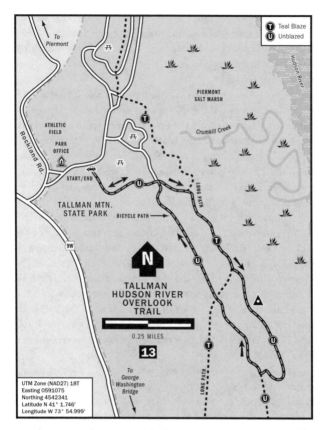

Teal Blaze
Unblazed

To Piermont

PIERMONT SALT MARSH

Hudson River

Crumkill Creek

ATHLETIC FIELD

PARK OFFICE

Rockland Rd.

START/END

TALLMAN MTN. STATE PARK

BICYCLE PATH →

LONG PATH

9W

N

TALLMAN HUDSON RIVER OVERLOOK TRAIL

0.25 MILES

13

To George Washington Bridge

LONG PATH

UTM Zone (NAD27) 18T
Easting 0591075
Northing 4542341
Latitude N 41° 1.746'
Longitude W 73° 54.999'

Tallman Mountain falls flatly in the middle of that debate. It came into existence in 1928, when the Palisades Interstate Park Commission appropriated 164 acres along the Palisades cliffs to keep them from being destroyed by industrial developers. Another 540 acres were added 14 years later. With the mountain having such a muscular-sounding soubriquet, might you expect something on the order of an 8-mile pinnacles hike or, at the very least, several hours of rock-scrambling capped by stupendous views?

Well, yes, but this is a different sort of state park, one that serves a multitude of interests, devoting much of its land to three picnic areas, a sports field and running track, basketball and tennis courts, and even a swimming pool (open from the third weekend in June through Labor Day).

Oh, did we forget to mention there is also hiking in Tallman? A section of the Long Path runs north–south through the entire length of the park and beyond. Overlapping a part of that is a 2.3-mile jaunt out to the bluffs and back, which some might argue is best described as a *walk*. Split the hairs however you like; this latter Hudson River Overlook Trail, while neither long nor strenuous, has a tremendous payoff in its unsurpassed bird's-eye view of the river and surrounding estuaries.

Look for the trailhead in the large parking area to the right of the park road, just past the office. From the middle of the lot's east side, stroll directly into the lush woodland, dense with sugar maples, black birches, and beeches. In about 0.25 miles, the somewhat rocky, hard-packed path crosses a paved bicycle lane. A hair under 100 yards beyond that is an intersection with the teal-blazed Long Path, which, if you follow it to the left, leads first to the swimming pools, then departs Tallman for Rockland Lake State Park and, continuing northward, Bear Mountain State Park.

Unless you are up for a highly ambitious hike or are feeling sweaty and in need of a dip, stay to the right. Though well trafficked, this stretch of trail feels fairly wild, with many stones protruding from the earth and an occasional tulip tree arching over the way. You may detect a bit of brininess to the air if the breeze is blowing from the east, but views of the Hudson are initially obscured, at least in summer, by the overgrowth crowding the path.

The vistas improve only after you break away from the Long Path in little more than a quarter mile, lunging left on an unblazed trail. The narrow passage descends slightly toward the marshland abutting the Hudson, fords a stream (dry in summer), then climbs gradually upward again, hopping from time to time over fallen trees. About 30 minutes into the hike, you'll reach a granite ledge that protrudes from the bluff several hundred feet above the Piermont salt marsh, providing an excellent vantage point from which to survey the Hudson River and its surroundings, including the Tappan Zee Bridge, far to the left, and the Piermont Pier. If you brought a pair of binoculars along, this is where you'll want to use them. It is also an ideal outpost for enjoying a sandwich.

Within a minute of leaving that viewpoint, where goldenrod and sumac color the understory, the trail forks; go right (west). Fewer than 100 paces should bring you to the cinder-covered multiuse track, where you again turn right. Follow this wide, easy path until, 30 paces after it morphs to pavement, you come to the spur you were on earlier that leads to the parking area. Take a left there to return to your car.

■ TO THE TRAILHEAD

Cross the George Washington Bridge and take the Palisades Interstate Parkway north to Exit 4. At the traffic light, turn left onto US 9W north and drive 2 miles to the park entrance on the right. The parking lot is beyond the park office, to the right.

14 Teatown Triple

■ OVERVIEW

LENGTH: 5 miles (including 1.1 miles for the Overlook Trail)

CONFIGURATION: Figure-eight, plus an additional loop for the Overlook Trail

SCENERY: Well-marked, gently rolling trails meander through shady forest of deciduous trees, laurel, and hemlock, around lake and a few swamps

EXPOSURE: Dense, protective canopy and only one open meadow

TRAFFIC: Light on Hidden Valley Trail across Blinn Road, but Lakeside Trail is quite popular on summer weekends

TRAIL SURFACE: Dirt, with occasional rocks and roots, and boardwalks

HIKING TIME: 2.5 hours

ACCESS: Dawn–dusk in summer; 9 a.m.–5 p.m. in winter; no fee; pets must be leashed; no bicycles

MAPS: At nature center; USGS Ossining

FACILITIES: Water and restrooms at nature center; picnic area, public phone

COMMENTS: For a fee, you may take a guided tour of Wildflower Island, a 2-acre sanctuary accessible via boardwalk. Open mid-April–September. Be sure to pre-register on weekends; call (914) 762-2912 for further details, or visit www.teatown.org.

■ SNAPSHOT

A lake with an island devoted to wildflowers, a couple of streams, and a number of boardwalks and bridges make this a can't-miss for family outings. The wild-at-heart should beat a path to the forested hillsides, too, where granite outcroppings, bogs, and meadows round out this diverse park. Teatown is crosscut by numerous paths, including a stretch of the Briarcliff–Peekskill Trail, so you can create as long or short a hike as fits your time or energy.

■ CLOSEUP

Some people feel that a hike is not complete without at least one animal sighting. A lone deer grazing on spruce needles, a fuzzy-tailed squirrel gathering acorns, even a swarm of bloodsucking mosquitoes in some intangible way validates the experience of being outdoors for a few hours. No hike comes with a guarantee,

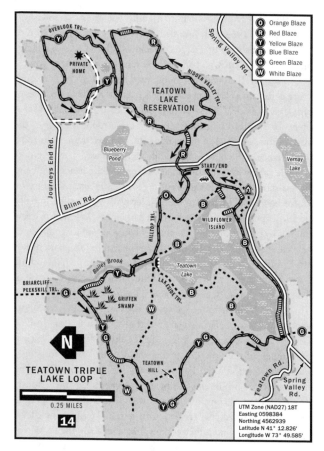

TEATOWN TRIPLE LAKE LOOP

Ⓞ	Orange Blaze
Ⓡ	Red Blaze
Ⓨ	Yellow Blaze
Ⓑ	Blue Blaze
Ⓖ	Green Blaze
Ⓦ	White Blaze

TEATOWN LAKE RESERVATION

PRIVATE HOME

OVERLOOK TRL.

Spring Valley Rd.

HIDDEN VALLEY TRL.

Blueberry Pond

Journeys End Rd.

Vernay Lake

START/END

Blinn Rd.

HILLTOP TRL.

WILDFLOWER ISLAND

Bailey Brook

Teatown Lake

BRIARCLIFF-PEEKSKILL TRL.

GRIFFEN SWAMP

LAKESIDE TRL.

N

TEATOWN HILL

Teatown Rd.

Spring Valley Rd.

0.25 MILES

14

UTM Zone (NAD27) 18T
Easting 0598384
Northing 4562939
Latitude N 41° 12.826'
Longitude W 73° 49.585'

of course, that a focus on things feral will come to fruition. But Teatown Lake does the next best thing, offering up a fail-safe selection of animals within its nature center.

Want to know what a corn snake looks like? The nature center has one, along with a black rat snake, a garter snake, tree frogs, a bearded dragon, a couple of ferrets, a bobcat, a coyote, a barn owl, and a moose. Well, okay, the last four are stuffed, but you get the idea: this is very much a family-friendly operation. Teatown was established in 1963 with just 190 acres, but it has since grown to 759 acres, consisting of a large lake and wildflower island, swampland, meadows, hardwood and conifer forests, and a craggy gorge.

Most of Teatown's highlights may be seen over three loops with a cumulative elevation gain of just over 1,000 feet and 5 miles of fairly easy walking. (These circuits may, of course, be tackled separately, for shorter excursions.) Two of these routes start near the road on the right side of the parking lot, and yes, there is indeed a good chance of encountering wildlife along the way. The trail forks as you leave the lot, with the orange-blazed Hilltop heading left and the red-slashed Hidden Valley cutting across the road. Keep to the left for now; you'll return to the Hidden Valley Trail later. Initially, the fairly open dirt track parallels the parking lot, followed in a few minutes by private dwellings to the right, in addition to a number of weather-stained erratics. From brushing by maples, shagbark hickories, hemlocks, and a handful of withered cedars, the path then shifts downhill through a shady patch of pines, arriving, near the base of that slope, at the north end of Teatown Lake.

Cross the concrete edge of the dam and then, after a short wooden walkway, hang a right onto the Northwest Trail (yellow tags). This gravel-lined track hugs Bailey Brook (more rocks than water much of the year) for perhaps 200 yards before crossing a bridge and continuing to the right, away from the lake. Diverging slowly from the brook, this northwest passage threads precariously through the moist, mucky Griffen Swamp (look for red cardinal flowers among the slippery rocks), with grass and ferns at ankle level and maple, beech, and tulip trees towering above. On the far side of a wooden span is a fork; stick with the yellow (now paired with green) blazes to the left. From there the meandering begins in earnest. On reaching a series of intersections, stride straight through the first junction (by the boardwalk), and bear right—still on yellow—at the next. Ten minutes of marching uphill should put you among laurels, hemlocks, and a mound of jagged granite.

Savor this setting, for in a few more steps you'll emerge on an open hillside under a nucleus of power lines. The climb continues in the shadow of those cables and their colossal support stanchions, with blueberry bushes, sassafras, Queen Anne's lace, and wild grapes thriving in the sun's strong glare. Stay to the left at the ensuing four-way intersection, and keep stomping up the steep, rock-filled slope. Finally at the top, canter left and descend on the other side of the power lines through knee- to waist-high grass and winged sumac. The yellow-green blazes veer off to the right at the base of one stanchion, finally bending away from those eyesores and back under a mantle of maples and oaks.

The trail shifts left at a stone wall, near a boggy patch, yielding in the process a pretty fair view of Teatown Lake. From there, it's downward by an imposing series of boulders, seemingly frozen in place as they were cascading down the hill. Turn right on the 20-foot-long boardwalk at the junction with the blue-blazed Lakeside Trail and, as soon as you've hit the west side of the lake, shift left (just before the road) onto a pontoon boardwalk that runs directly over a section of the water. This segment of the hike rewards your decision to bring field specs, as the birding is typically excellent, and it is easy to whittle time off the clock counting mallards, swans, and Canada geese (and occasionally something more exotic).

When you've tired of birding, press onward through the shady nook by the shore, over the next span, and into a second maple-graced recess. Moving east by the water, lope left at the wooden stairs to the nature center and pass over the boardwalk. Stroll by the enormous tulip tree, go straight across the trail junction (left leads down a boardwalk to a view of Wildflower Island through a bird blind), then veer right off the blue trail to return to the parking area.

Once more at the trailhead by the road, this time follow the red blazes of the Hidden Valley Trail (HV) across the asphalt for an entirely different look at the park. Proceed through the gap in the wall and over the boardwalk, into a grassy, fern-speckled meadow, with an apple orchard on one side, black walnut trees on the other, and a handful of dogwoods, maples, and sycamores tossed in for good measure. Shuffle right at the four-way junction and remain with the red blazes throughout the entire 1.6-mile loop, seeing along the way thick clusters of pines and hemlocks, several dramatic escarpments, and even another boardwalk by an extended marsh.

The yellow-blazed spur of the Overlook Trail (OT) surfaces a couple of minutes past an impressively high granite formation. If your soles still have good spring, consider adding this 1.1-mile mini-loop to the tour: it leads to one of the park's more untamed areas, where the rough-cut beauty is highly appealing and the flush of wildflowers in the spring and summer adds to its allure. From the short series of stone steps that lead away from the HV, the path ascends to a small reed-rimmed pond, its muddy banks blooming with lobelia in summer. Continue to the right, over additional steps, making use of the guide rope as you climb. Take a moment to catch your breath, meanwhile enjoying, in the break of the rock formations to the right, the great view of the swamp you passed through earlier, and the tree-lined hills beyond; the trail snakes higher still, but the vistas won't get any better. The next set of steps heralds the summit, and the highest point of the hike, at 584 feet. The wild look to the woods here, with lichen-speckled rocks scattered among maples, oaks, birches, and mountain laurel, suggests a deeply forested wilderness—even though there's a house tucked just out of sight below the crest. That illusion dissipates rapidly as the OT descends to a paved driveway, where a couple of monster homes are visible to the right. Swing left on the asphalt, and in 50 paces head right, returning to the shelter of the trees. Back at the pond, retrace your steps to the turnoff from the HV, then veer right, once more following the red blazes. Stay with those markings all the way to the meadow, and from there to the parking lot.

■ TO THE TRAILHEAD

From the Saw Mill Parkway take the exit for the Taconic Parkway north. Get off the Taconic at the NY 134/Ossining exit, turning left onto NY 134/Kitchawan Road. Drive 0.25 miles and turn right on Spring Valley Road. In 0.8 miles bear right on Blinn Road and continue 0.1 mile to the lakeside parking lot on the left.

15 Walt Whitman Sampler

■ OVERVIEW

LENGTH: 3.6 miles	**ACCESS:** Year-round, dawn–dusk; $2 for Suffolk County residents, $5 for tourists Memorial Day–Labor Day, free rest of year; no bicycles on most trails; pets must be leashed
CONFIGURATION: Loop	
SCENERY: Rolling, mixed deciduous forest hiding a quiet pond, gnarly laurel thickets, and Long Island's highest point	
	MAPS: At Walt Whitman Birthplace; Long Island Greenbelt Trail Conference; USGS Huntington
EXPOSURE: Lush canopy protection	
TRAIL SURFACE: Dirt, roots, and pebbles	**FACILITIES:** Restrooms, water, public phone, and playground at picnic area
TRAFFIC: Light on weekdays, can get really busy on weekends	**COMMENTS:** Riding stables are right behind the picnic area. For information, call (631) 351-9168.
HIKING TIME: 2 hours	

■ SNAPSHOT

The seaside vistas are overgrown from when Walt Whitman roamed this historic woodland, but the densely forested hills still provide a poetic setting for a short hike. A labyrinth of trails snakes by a picturesque pond amid laurels, white pines, and rhododendrons— as well as a full complement of hardwoods—on the way to Jayne's Hill, the highest point on Long Island.

■ CLOSEUP

"West Hills is a romantic and beautiful spot. It is the most hilly and elevated part of Long Island . . . afford[ing] an extensive and pleas- ant view," Walt Whitman wrote in 1850 of the hills that rise above his boyhood home. In Whitman's day it was possible to view the Connecticut shore from atop the highest peak, Jayne's Hill, and watch schooners sailing by Fire Island to the south. Those vistas are gone now—overgrown by mountain laurel, beech, and birch

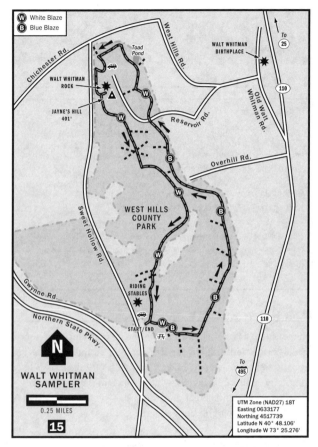

White Blaze
Blue Blaze

To 25

Chichester Rd.

West Hills Rd.

Toad Pond

WALT WHITMAN BIRTHPLACE

WALT WHITMAN ROCK

JAYNE'S HILL 401'

Reservoir Rd.

110

Old Walt Whitman Rd.

Overhill Rd.

WEST HILLS COUNTY PARK

Sweet Hollow Rd.

Gwynne Rd.

RIDING STABLES

Northern State Pkwy.

START/END

110

To 495

N

WALT WHITMAN SAMPLER

0.25 MILES

15

UTM Zone (NAD27) 18T
Easting 0633177
Northing 4517739
Latitude N 40° 48.106'
Longitude W 73° 25.276'

trees—but this remains a delightful place, no less hilly and inspiring today than it once was to one of our country's great poets.

In 1825, when Silas Wood, an early historian of Long Island, had "High Hill" surveyed, its top crested at 354 feet of elevation. While paltry by western standards, that was enough to rank this mount as highest on the island. Its name was later changed to Jayne's Hill, after the family that lived here, and having been resurveyed a number of times since, it now officially tops out at 400.9 feet above sea level.

This meandering hike traverses the colorful forests of the West Hills, crossing the top of Jayne's Hill about halfway out. There are many maverick bike and bridle trails intersecting your route, but the main path is well blazed and fairly easy to follow. Begin at the far side of the picnic grounds, by the edge of the woods. Keep to the right, walking toward the fenced field and looking for white blazes on the trees. Stay with those as the markings glide to the left side of the sports field–cum–dog-walking area. Once you're past the corner of the fence, you'll find a blue-blazed path to the left. Turn there and then turn left again onto the sandy bridle path. Stick with the blue blazes as they veer right at the fork, then right once more in another ten steps. Now drifting among birches, oaks, and an occasional dogwood—to say nothing of scads of mountain laurel—the well-indicated, pebbly track shifts left at a T. It then passes a number of spurs as it ascends steadily to higher ground, swinging left in three minutes at the T-junction with a bridle trail. For hikers with a good sense of orientation, the many side trails in this forest offer great bushwhacking possibilities.

In due time, the clearly blazed trail loops to the left of a gray house. About a minute later, it meets a wide crossing with another bridle path, where it continues straight ahead, single file, until it merges with a horse track: pivot left there. Bear left once more at the next broad fork, away from the private dwellings. With laurels now the trail's dominant plant, the blue blazes swerve sharply right off the main route in 150 feet, adhering closely to a ridgeline. Head right when you hit the T with a bridle path, and a couple of minutes after passing a horse stable to the right, just beyond the park boundary, you will come to a set of erosion-control steps.

Access to Jayne's Hill is atop that staircase. Instead of following the road, though, stroll across the pavement, picking up the white blazes on its opposite side, near a chain-link fence. With that barrier to the right, and white pines towering overhead, you have now started the more enjoyable half of the hike. On reaching a small rise, the path descends sharply away from the majestic conifers, into a beech- and birch-shaded gully. The trail levels off briefly, trots right at a fork, goes right at the ensuing crossing, then dives down-hill again among a green carpet of Canada mayflowers. The white blazes lead left at the succeeding fork, and a few paces beyond is Toad Pond. Though marred by a metal fence stretched over its right end, this is an attractive (albeit gradually silting up) body of water, shaped like a crooked, elongated smile.

Ignore the steps that lead away from the pond and proceed along its boggy bank. The track runs beside a bog for the next sev-eral yards and can be quite wet in spring, but soon the ground grows steadily steeper, plugging upward toward Jayne's Hill. It requires only a minute to get by the most precipitous part of that climb, one breathtaking, heart-pounding minute. After that the elevation gain is more gradual, almost imperceptible, until you heave to the left on the bridle path, and in a few dozen strides the trail ends at the Jayne's Hill parking lot.

Hug the right side of the lot, circling around a pine tree and hewing hard to the right of the swing set and dilapidated latrine. Stick with this wide, white-blazed track, which is lined with lavender-flowering myrtle, dogwood, and oak, as it cruises to the right at the subsequent fork and left at the one after that. The terrain grows more lush with every step you take, with mountain laurel, white pine, and black birch creeping back into the forested mix. The top of Jayne's Hill lies just ahead, a site marked by two benches, a rock with a plaque, and a pale-blue water tower. Second-growth trees now block out the view that Whitman enjoyed from this, the highest ground on Long Island, but you may still derive pleasure from the tranquility of the spot, as well as the Whitman quote on the plaque.

Continue to the right of the rock, down several steps through an overgrown tangle of brier, chokeberry, and poison ivy. The trail levels off among ferns and oaks, then rolls with the undulating texture of the hillside. This pleasantly secluded, moss-sided track ends at a split-rail fence, where you scoot right onto a bridle path. In 45 yards, at a four-way crossing, the white-blazed trail scuttles left, descending through brier, maple, birch, and cedar, and then crosses another four-way intersection. From a leveling off, the path rises negligibly, culminating in a left turn at a T. Go left at the sub-sequent fork, and with the white blazes clearly visible, hang a right at the next major turn, in about 25 feet. Some 100 yards later, the track diverges to the right—then left, in 30 paces—and, having descended briefly, darts through a narrow livestock barrier.

You remain on this ridge for a while, slightly above the trees of the surrounding hills, as rhododendron makes a surprise appear-ance, blanketing the sides of the slope. A further descent over log steps leads to a second barrier. Once you're through that, the white blazes shift left, crossing the bridle path and slipping through a rail fence (look for spotted wintergreen in springtime). After a few min-utes of walking, you should see the roof of the riding stables on the right. A short descent follows, delivering you to yet another set of rails. The horse trails trot left, right, and straight ahead, with your route running between the right and straight options. A few furlongs more and the path ends, dropping you off by the picnic grounds, with the parking lot directly beyond.

If you have time to spare before or after the hike, plan to visit the nearby Walt Whitman Birthplace State Historic Site. Displays in this recently renovated, early-19th-century farmhouse, at 246 Old Walt Whitman Road, include portraits of Whitman, his poetry, letters, a tape recording of his voice, and more. Call (631) 427-5240 for details, or visit www.waltwhitman.org.

■ TO THE TRAILHEAD

Follow the Long Island Expressway (I-495) east and take Exit 42, merging onto the Northern State Parkway east. Leave the parkway at Exit 40S and drive 0.2 miles south on Walt Whitman Road (NY 110). Turn right on Old Country Road and continue 0.3 miles, then go right again on Sweet Hollow Road. Proceed 0.5 miles to the parking lot and picnic area on the right.

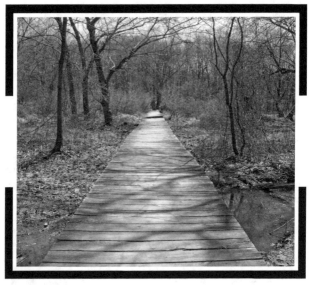

Wooden boardwalks encourage hikers to explore the swamps in Cheesequake State Park.

Nearby New Jersey

16 *Cheesequake Natural Area Trail*

■ OVERVIEW

LENGTH: 5.5 miles

CONFIGURATION: Loop

SCENERY: Sandy pine barrens, humid freshwater swamps connected by boardwalks, and lush hardwood forests boasting some of area's tallest trees

EXPOSURE: Mostly shady

TRAIL SURFACE: Dirt, roots, sand

TRAFFIC: It can get rather hectic May–September, especially on weekends

HIKING TIME: 3 hours

ACCESS: Year-round, 8 a.m.–dusk; Memorial Day weekend–Labor Day, $5 weekdays, $10 weekends; free

Tuesdays and rest of year; $50 parks pass gives access to all New Jersey state parks for one calendar year

MAPS: At park office and interpretive center; USGS South Amboy

FACILITIES: Restrooms, water, and telephone at park office; interpretive nature center, campground, picnic areas, playground

COMMENTS: The attractive interpretive center is accessible by foot and offers educational exhibits and activities. Call (732) 566-3208 for information, or visit www.state.nj.us/dep/parksand forests/parks/cheesequake.html.

■ SNAPSHOT

If you enjoy traipsing through cedar swamps and backwoods bayous while bounding over boardwalks, Cheesequake is for you. The state park is well endowed in each of those categories, with plenty of raw, natural beauty to appeal to other tastes. The birding is great by its lake and marshlands. Then there are several notable forests, populated by stands of monumental oaks, tulip trees, and white pines. And the wide, swiftly flowing Cheesequake Creek is so alluring you may be tempted to portage your own canoe.

■ CLOSEUP

For most people, Cheesequake State Park is little more than a green spot on the road map, with the Garden State Parkway cutting across it like a bull charging through a red-ribbon fence. On

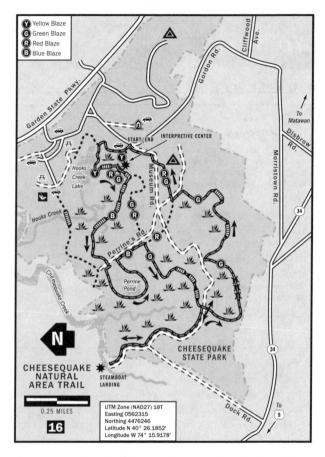

the way to or from the Big Apple, few motorists give the slightest thought to stopping. That's their loss, because this 1,274-acre park is extravagantly beautiful, partly because it straddles a transitional zone between two major ecosystems. Miles of trails (and a hefty number of boardwalks) meander among pine barrens, a cedar swamp, marshlands, and open fields. In fact, there is so much eye candy in this diverse terrain that at the end of a day of hiking, many trekkers don't want to leave—so they set up a tent and camp.

Cheesequake, incidentally, is not a phonetic misspelling of some heavy dairy-based dessert. Back in June 1940, when the preserve was first opened to the public, park officials plucked the word from the language of the Lenape Indians, who hunted and fished these grounds into the 1700s before being wiped out by white settlers. The Lenapes were but the last in a long line of Indian tribes who found the Cheesequake (properly—if seldom—pronounced CHESS-quick) area inviting, with the earliest traces of occupation dating back 5,000 years.

The trailhead and map kiosk are to the far left of the parking area. Head out on the wide path and turn right at the fork, in 150 feet, onto the Yellow Trail, where blueberry bushes and sassafras compose the understory and maples, mountain laurel, and various oaks provide shade. Bear left at the slanted T, as the moss-sided track hugs a ridgeline that tapers toward Hooks Creek Lake. Enjoy the vantage point high over the water, which is attractively framed by pitch pines, cattails, and other reeds. On descending the wooden staircase, continue to the left, as Yellow draws you to the side of a salt marsh, where cormorants, snowy egrets, pine warblers, and other shore birds may lurk in the cover of salt hay and cord grass. From there the path arcs to the right and hits a boardwalk, bringing you to a freshwater flood plain (another fine place for birding).

Take the right fork to the interpretive center. In walking under the wooden archway, crossing a bridge, and steering toward the wood-sided pavilion, exchange yellow blazes for red and green ones; then pick up the Blue Trail to the right of the building, and stay with it along the spine of the ridge.

Once again back at marsh level, the path meets a boardwalk, with a stream running under it. Go right at the T atop the stairs that follow, sticking with Blue as it diverges from the red and green blazes. Then it is down another set of stairs, over a short boardwalk (surrounded by an attractive swamp), and up some more steps. On stomping down yet another set of stairs, the marsh will now be on either side of you, as the track morphs into a five-foot-wide boardwalk.

Atop the next staircase Blue jogs right, overlooking the marsh, then left, adhering to the contours of a ridge. Ignore the traces as the path dips again toward the marshland, sticking with the blue discs. After puttering left, the path delivers you to an unpaved road, where you slip under the wooden arch and hang a right, followed by a quick left, still on Blue as it overlaps a wide, sandy forest road. Check out the bird blind on the left, where you may spy on black-crested cormorants, ducks, and gulls on Perrine Pond; then, on continuing along the path, don't forget to scan the sky for osprey swooping over the marsh to the right. Swallows also tend to mingle among the reeds, and in the loamy ground to the left, as the now-gravel-surfaced track pulls away from the water, you may be able to discern the freshly burrowed holes of fox dens. At the T with a second woods road, bear right, and in two to three minutes veer right on the Green Trail.

The path initially clings to a ridge when it departs the gravel road, before dropping to a swamp speckled green with ferns and skunk cabbage. A boardwalk here stretches for a whopping 100 yards, ending at a wooden staircase. Tread up that, then down the steps that follow, onto the next boardwalk, surrounded suddenly, marvelously, by cedar trees. The walkway snakes through this cedar swamp, where the water has been dyed orange by tree tannins leaching into the underlying soil. The planks end briefly—keep to the right—only to resume for a short spell. Then it's briskly uphill, back among laurels and oaks.

On hitting the park road, you have three choices: proceed directly across on Green, swing right for Steamboat Landing, or lurch left for an early bailout. The detour to Steamboat Landing is highly scenic and requires only about a half hour for the round-trip. As the conifers growing on the embankment to the left and right of the dirt road give way to hardwood trees, peer left, about 70 yards in, for one of the park's largest white oaks. After coming abreast of a marsh, the lane forks: dogleg left around the barrier and make an immediate right onto Dock Road. In three minutes, the unpaved lane dead-ends at a bend in Cheesequake Creek, by a confluence of streams, with the rotting pilings of an old steamboat landing 70 feet across the swiftly flowing water. There is a subtle serenity to this delightful spot that makes it well worth visiting, with an osprey-nesting platform, installed in 2007, an additional attraction.

Back at the four-way intersection, venture right on an extension of Green. As you shuffle along, check out the spectacular stand of white pines, primarily to the left. Too soon you leave that behind and ascend a slight slope that is well scarred with roots, followed by a wooden staircase. Green dips again shortly and meanders over three bridges, then bends left by some wooden rails. In time, the path approaches Museum Road, only to swerve right just before meeting it.

The ensuing segment of the hike showcases a few kettle-hole depressions to the right, and in the swamp on the left an impressive grove of tulip trees, many quite monumental. Green soon arcs left toward the heart of that swamp and slips over 175 feet of boardwalk, jumping to the left at the end of the planks. After treading through a deeply rutted patch, look to the right for a giant beech tree, an icon among the many hardwoods in the area.

The group-camping area is directly ahead when you pass under the wooden arch. Instead of entering it, go left on the paved road, and in a couple of minutes scamper right, under the next archway. The Red Trail joins Green here, holding to the back of the campground and scooting left as it approaches the second camping field. Mosey right on the paved Museum Road and, remaining with that, return to the parking area.

■ TO THE TRAILHEAD

Take Exit 120 off the Garden State Parkway south and make a right onto Laurence Harbor Parkway, then another right, in 0.25 miles, onto Cliffwood Avenue. At the T, turn right onto Gordon Road and continue 0.6 miles to the park entrance. The park office is on the right. The trailhead parking area is the next lot on the left.

High Mountain Summit Loop

■ OVERVIEW

LENGTH: 6.1 miles	**HIKING TIME:** 3 hours
CONFIGURATION: Balloon	**ACCESS:** Year-round, dawn–dusk; no fee, pets must be leashed, no horseback riding
SCENERY: Rolling trail snakes through dense woodlands and lush wetlands that harbor endangered plants and a traprock glade	**MAPS:** USGS Paterson; visit www.hike leader.com/highmountainpark.htm or www.waynetownship.com/maps/ mountainpark.pdf
EXPOSURE: Generous shade until the summit, which is very open	
TRAIL SURFACE: Rock-packed dirt, loose stones, some grassy patches	**FACILITIES:** None
TRAFFIC: Often on the light side, but a favorite getaway of students from nearby William Patterson University	**COMMENTS:** Heavy spring rains may transform trails into cascading streams. For further information, call the Wayne Township Department of Parks and Recreation: 973-694-1800, ext. 3260.

■ SNAPSHOT

The run up High Mountain is a great workout, vacuuming the air out of your lungs. The view of Manhattan from the grass-and-granite-graced peak is breathtaking, too, but there's more, including a small cascade, numerous stream crossings, a romantic pond, remote swamp hollows—even some Paleolithic rock shelters concealed in a ravine.

■ CLOSEUP

High Mountain Park, a 1,154-acre Nature Conservancy preserve, is a good news/bad news sort of place. First, the bad news: many of the trails in this attractive sanctuary have been terribly eroded by ATVs and dirt bikes. As for the good news: this is one of the most beautiful parcels of land in the entire New Jersey Piedmonts, with the hike rising to a bald peak from which the Manhattan skyline is boldly visible, and dropping down through a hardwood forest and fertile swamp. There are also several prehistoric rock shelters in

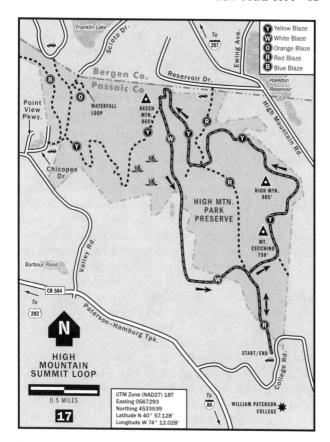

Franklin Lake

Scioto Dr.

To 287

Ewing Ave.

Y Yellow Blaze
W White Blaze
O Orange Blaze
R Red Blaze
B Blue Blaze

Bergen Co.
Passaic Co.

Reservoir Dr.

Haledon
Reservoir

Point
View
Pkwy.

WATERFALL
LOOP

BEECH
MTN.
869'

High Mountain Rd.

Chicopee
Dr.

HIGH MTN.
PARK
PRESERVE

HIGH MTN.
885'

Barbour Pond

Valley Rd.

MT.
CECCHINO
750'

CR 504

To 202

Paterson–Hamburg Tpk.

START/END

College Rd.

N

**HIGH
MOUNTAIN
SUMMIT
LOOP**

0.5 MILES

17

UTM Zone (NAD27) 18T
Easting 0567293
Northing 4533539
Latitude N 40° 57.128'
Longitude W 74° 12.028'

To 80

WILLIAM PATERSON
COLLEGE

the vicinity, and in more recent times a few of the ridge tops were used during the Revolutionary War to light signal beacons.

Pick up the Red Trail on the right side of the relatively new trailhead parking lot, on the opposite side of College Road from William Paterson University (this lot is indicated by a green sign emblazoned with HIGH MOUNTAIN PARK in gold lettering). Don't worry about the gravelly ground, as it's all uphill from here (your cumulative elevation gain is 975 feet), with Red breaking left just ahead, into the shelter of chestnut oak, black birch, and maple. In less than a minute Red turns left again, momentarily following a well-grooved track before departing the rutted route, jumping left at a sizable, graffiti-scarred erratic. Remain with the red blazes as a minor descent commences, then turn left at a T, in about 50 feet. As is typical of this undulating terrain, an ascent soon ensues; ignore the unblazed spurs, scooting right onto the yellow-blazed trail during a brief lull in the uphill slog.

After initially rising for perhaps as little as 30 steps, Yellow branches right at a fork, rock-hops over a swamp stream, and continues gently descending as it meanders farther right. It then veers left at a deeply grooved rut, accumulating altitude for just a minute before resuming a slight downward trend. Ignore the many maverick side trails and swing right, still with Yellow, at the next major bifurcation. On descending still farther and skidding by a couple more spurs, the path finally begins to gain ground, carrying you over a hardy volume of marble- and cueball-size rocks.

High Mountain tops out at 885 feet, with most of the gain achieved on the drive to the parking lot. Even so, count on a five- to ten-minute ascent on Yellow, before the wide track levels off and then starts losing ground. Stay with the yellow blazes, dead-on, at the four-way intersection. Your ascent resumes when you cruise left at the T a minute later, with the path alternating between pebbles and bedrock. The terrain near the crest, colored by oak, black birch, sarsaparilla, and spicebush, is honeycombed with the deep ruts of dirt bikers, with all roads leading to the top.

Stick with the yellow markings to the exposed peak of High Mountain, where buttercups and purple violets grow and the Manhattan skyline is vibrantly visible on a clear day. The grooved stone under your feet, by the way, is an unusual form of basaltic traprock that the Nature Conservancy describes as globally imperiled—whether by too incessant an application of spray paint by vandals or the spinning tires of dirt bikes, we're not sure. Moving along, glide right on leaving the vista point and rejoin the forest road. Steer to the left of the large oak when you come to the lush opening in the trees, and follow the yellow blazes to the next rise. This is a wonderful section of the highland forest and a fun ramble through several pocket meadows, where deer often graze and the interplay of grass and rocks contributes considerably to the eye appeal.

Soon enough a downhill stretch commences, drawing you back into the cover of the forest. From initially adhering to the rocky forest road, the trail darts left, at a pause in that descent, narrowing to single file within an overgrown corridor of maple, oak, and birch. Check out the spur to the right; it ends by a scenic glade where a head-high glacial erratic abuts the stream.

Surging straight at the subsequent junction, the path hops over that same stream. A minute later, there is a four-way intersection with the red-blazed trail you were on earlier. If you are not good at orienteering, jump left onto Red and return to the trailhead. Otherwise, take the middle option and hew to the right at the fork directly after, still with the yellow markings. Yellow meanders along a ridge for a spell, then begins to lose elevation, bottoming out in a hemlock-and-cedar swamp, where it hairpins sharply left. (The trace to the right, also sporting yellow blazes, ends at a road in less than 100 feet.)

Here begins a route-finding challenge, as the yellow markings have—as of our last two outings—been mysteriously blacked out. Basically, when the path meets the rock-filled swamp, it swoops straight across (look for the dark swatches on the trees where the yellow markings once were) and soars up the opposite hill. A couple of yellow blazes resurface just before you hit a forest road, where you merge left. In about a minute, this lane meets a junction with a white-blazed trail, which you follow straight on, as Yellow (its markings still obliterated) branches right. Even with many of the initial white blazes also effaced, this is a fairly clear and easy track to follow.

The spring display of wildflowers on High Mountain is divine, but you pay for that pulchritude on this stretch, which resembles an active arroyo in wet weather. In spite of such soggy conditions, you are more likely to see deer and squirrels here than muskrats and otters. As you move downhill, ignore the forest road that emerges from a field of traprock shale on the right. Having drifted through a slate-lined gully, where ramps and trout lily thrive by the side of a seasonal stream, White breaks right momentarily, departing the forest road only to return to the wide track in a few minutes. Soon the white blazes hop left, over the wide stream, and then swerve right and arrive (via a short spur, also to the right) at a romantic pond, with chestnut oak and black birch bracketing the idyllic scene.

Back on the main trail, bear right at the fork and rock-hop over the wash, staying with the blazes as they cut left, neatly avoiding a golf course. Yes, you read correctly: for the next several minutes, the path skirts the perimeter of the North Jersey Country Club and passes behind a few impressive rock formations. Shortly after the golf course, keep left at the fork, still with White. It's uphill from here, with a couple of stream crossings and a vine-covered cabin ruin thrown in for the sake of variety. Much of the ascent overlaps what appears to be a sluice of an old streambed, with its broken-up surface providing enough friction under the feet to encourage an appointment with Dr. Scholl.

Check out the bluff of traprock to the left, which extends for more than 40 feet and rises an impressive 25 feet: that depression near its base may be the remains of a Paleolithic shelter. White ends at a fork a couple of minutes later, as you pick up red blazes and continue straight. In bypassing the yellow-blazed route on the left, you have completed the loop. Remain with Red all the way back to College Road.

■ TO THE TRAILHEAD

Leave I-80 at Exit 53 onto NJ 23 north, and after 1.3 miles turn right onto Alps Road. Continue 2.8 miles, then swing right onto the Hamburg Turnpike/CR 504. After the intersection with Valley Road, drive 1.1 miles and turn left on College Road. Proceed for 0.6 miles to the parking lot on the left.

18 Norvin Green's High Point

■ OVERVIEW

LENGTH: 3 miles

CONFIGURATION: Balloon loop

SCENERY: Steep, densely forested climb to stellar 360-degree panoramas revealing New York City skyline

EXPOSURE: Very shady, except on the bald High Point and neighboring ridge

TRAIL SURFACE: Rock-filled dirt, loose stones, and bedrock on summit ridge

TRAFFIC: Can be light, except at High Point, which is usually rather crowded

HIKING TIME: 2 hours

ACCESS: Year-round, 9 a.m.–dusk; no fee; no bicycles, no motorized vehicles

MAPS: At kiosk by Weis Ecology Center; USGS Wanaque

FACILITIES: Nature center, water, restrooms, and public telephone at Weis Ecology Center

COMMENTS: Rain-fed streams may make some water crossings tough. Remember to bring a flashlight if you want to go spelunking in the old mines. For further information, call (973) 962-7031, or visit www.njparks andforests.org/parks/norvin.html.

■ SNAPSHOT

If you're feeling adventurous, you had best dust off your sturdiest hiking boots before trekking into Norvin Green. This is a moderately demanding hike into an undeveloped, seriously rugged locale, with the reward for your effort being a mountaintop vista, a historic mine, and nonstop natural beauty.

■ CLOSEUP

Norvin Green is an undeveloped park, and our loop is more physically demanding than many others in this guide. Yet this hike should be within the abilities of all but the most tender-footed of readers. (For a more challenging outing, see the Norvin Green entry in this book's companion volume, *60 Hikes within 60 Miles: New York City*.)

To find the trailhead, cut to the north side of the parking lot and cross the narrow footbridge. Take an immediate left, shy of the

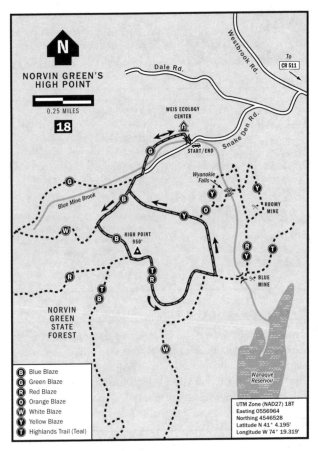

NORVIN GREEN'S
HIGH POINT

0.25 MILES

18

WEIS ECOLOGY
CENTER

START/END

Dale Rd.

Westbrook Rd.

To
CR 511

Snake Den Rd.

Wyanokie
Falls

ROOMY
MINE

Blue Mine Brook

HIGH POINT
950'

BLUE
MINE

NORVIN
GREEN
STATE
FOREST

Wanaque
Reservoir

B Blue Blaze
G Green Blaze
R Red Blaze
O Orange Blaze
W White Blaze
Y Yellow Blaze
T Highlands Trail (Teal)

UTM Zone (NAD27) 18T
Easting 0556964
Northing 4546528
Latitude N 41° 4.195'
Longitude W 74° 19.319'

concrete picnic tables, and stick with the pine-shaded path, heading west and marked with green blazes. By the time you reach the northwest corner of Highlands Natural Pool (HNP), on the left, those markings will have been joined by two others: an orange L in a white circle and a green W in a white square, the latter denoting the Weis Trail. All three blazes branch left at the fork here; follow them, keeping to the west side of the HNP.

Stick with the green blazes as the rock-strewn path crosses a couple of bridges and ascends above the HNP; both the L and W trails eventually diverge. This circuitous route, which seems to follow a vestigial streambed under a canopy of black birch, oak, and maple trees, comes to a kiosk at a junction with a forest road. Instead of following the green tags to the right, step behind the kiosk and switch to the blue-blazed Hewitt Butler Trail (which overlaps the yellow-dotted white-circle blazes for a time), as the uphill slog resumes.

In a few minutes, once the rock-strewn trail has scratched through a laurel patch and reached a minor crest, the yellow dots break left—remain with Hewitt Butler straight ahead. A slight dip is followed by another false summit, atop lichen-speckled bedrock, with great views to the west. Studded with pitch pine and scrub oak, this is an ideal picnic spot, as is a second picturesque nook (highlighted by a huge erratic) at the next summit, just up the trail.

Shortly after the path veers left off the crest, it arrives at a junction with a white-blazed trail, on the right. Hew to the left, still with Hewitt Butler, and continue the down–up progress of the ridgeline, passing among further blueberry bushes, pitch pines, pin oaks, laurels, and, throughout the wetter weeks of the summer and early autumn, an amazing assortment of mushrooms. Take a left at the next intersection, abandoning the blue blazes for the red-dotted white circles of the Wyanokie Circular Trail (Wyanokie); you'll also join the Highlands Trail (teal diamonds) here. A final rock scramble out of this nest of laurels delivers you to the top of High Point.

To merely say that High Point summit is granite bedrock partly clad in grass, fringed with knee-high ferns, blueberry bushes, and such wildflowers as Indian strawberry and goats beard is to do its beauty an injustice. Even with a cluster of spicebush and pitch pines at the periphery, the view here at 950 feet is spectacular, a 360-degree panorama that lists among its highlights I-287 to the south, and the New York City skyline beyond that. Your (reluctant) descent from this idyllic dome begins on its east side. The downhill slope—which yields a great glimpse of Wanaque Reservoir—begins in earnest as you put the stand of dead chestnuts, a field of boulders and, in summer, a broad swath of goldenrod and purple pokeweed, behind you.

Near the trough, as Wyanokie approaches a stream gully, the white-blazed Post Brook Trail commences on the right. Bear left, remaining with Wyanokie, and rock-hop over the stream. At the next intersection you'll find the other end of the trail that branched off earlier from the Hewitt Butler, marked with yellow-dotted white circles. Turn left here to commence the return leg of the hike. If time and energy permit, however, consider traipsing a short distance farther along Wyanokie, across the footbridge, to the Blue Mine, where the broad Blue Mine Brook flows into its yawning orifice, and frogs and birds bathe in the eddying current. The Blue Mine, known variously since it opened in 1765 as the London, Whynokie, and Iron Hill mine, derives its current moniker from the bluish hue of its iron ore.

Alternatively, as you resume the climb on the yellow-dotted trail, you can make another colorful side trip: to the right is an orange-tagged track, marked by a wooden post that indicates the way to Roomy Mine and Falls. The top of the waterfall, at 550 feet, is worth the detour in its own right, as the great cascade tumbles into a jumble of oversize boulders. Beyond that is Roomy Mine, named after Benjamin Roome, a 19th-century surveyor.

As you continue along the yellow-dotted route, the steepness of the path soon moderates as it passes a highly scenic series of rocky protrusions and uplift, boulders and bedrock that herald your imminent right turn back onto the Hewitt Butler. From this familiar juncture, retrace your steps to the trailhead.

■ TO THE TRAILHEAD

Take Exit 57 off I-287 onto Skyline Drive, Ringwood direction. Drive north 5 miles to the stop sign and turn left on Erskine Road. Proceed 0.1 mile to Greenwood Lake Turnpike (CR 511) and make a left, followed by a right—in 1.7 miles—onto Westbrook Road. Drive 1.4 miles, then veer left at the fork and turn left onto Snake Den Road in another 0.5 miles. Proceed 0.7 miles, past the large parking area on the right (just after the purple Quonset hut), and turn left at the fork, by the sign for the Weis Ecology Center. Make an immediate right into the parking lot.

OVERVIEW

LENGTH: 4.5 miles	**MAPS:** Posted at kiosk and available at Darlington County Park, 600 Darlington Avenue, Mahwah, (973) 327-3500; www.co.bergen.nj.us/bcparks/LocalParks.aspx (select Ramapo Valley from the drop down list, then scroll down and click Ramapo Reservation Trails); USGS Wanaque
CONFIGURATION: Loop	
SCENERY: Lush forests, historic ruins, placid lake, scenic streams, many rock outcroppings	
EXPOSURE: Dense canopy sometimes interrupted by open, grassy spots along the lake	
TRAIL SURFACE: Dirt, rocks, roots	**FACILITIES:** Parking lot has kiosk with posted map, public phone, and portable toilet
TRAFFIC: Light–moderate; Ramapo Lake circuit is hugely popular on weekends	
	COMMENTS: Nearby Campgaw Mountain County Reservation and Ramapo Valley County Reservation offer great camping. Permits can be obtained at Darlington County Park (see above). For further information, call (973) 962-7031, or visit www.njparksandforests.org/parks/ramapo.html.
HIKING TIME: 2.5 hours	
ACCESS: Year-round, 8 a.m.–8 p.m.; no fee; bicycles prohibited on most trails, no motorized vehicles	

SNAPSHOT

This trek has so much diversity you'll hardly feel the time pass. In addition to a scenic lake, a towering bluff, and glacial erratics by the bushel, these woods are inundated with wildlife (including black bears), birds beyond count, and a spring flower display that a horticulturalist would envy.

CLOSEUP

There are so many trails tattooed into the hills of the Ramapo Mountains, it is sometimes hard to know where to begin. The following hike, interspersed with glacial uplift, an expansive lake, a few picturesque streams, and a far-reaching vista, serves as a colorful introduction to the Ramapo Mountains. (For a more challenging

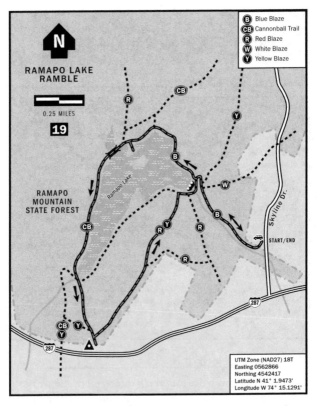

RAMAPO LAKE RAMBLE

0.25 MILES

19

RAMAPO MOUNTAIN STATE FOREST

Ramapo Lake

Skyline Dr.

START/END

287

B	Blue Blaze
CB	Cannonball Trail
R	Red Blaze
W	White Blaze
Y	Yellow Blaze

UTM Zone (NAD27) 18T
Easting 0562866
Northing 4542417
Latitude N 41° 1.9473'
Longitude W 74° 15.1291'

jaunt of 16-plus miles, refer to this book's companion volume, *60 Hikes within 60 Miles: New York City*.)

From your car, walk to the southwest corner of the large parking area, in the direction of the kiosk and portable toilet, and follow the wide, blue-blazed MacEvoy Trail (MT) as it passes between the remnants of an old foundation. Steer to the right at the first fork, by a small cascade (look for the bright-yellow blossoms of Jerusalem artichoke from mid- to late summer), sticking with the blue blazes as they lead you upward. Go right again, in about one minute, at the next fork; it's an easy scramble over granite bedrock. Bear left at the subsequent intersection, holding to the MT as the hard track levels off and meets the white-blazed Todd Trail. Shortly after crossing a seasonal stream, the path rises again and then, in a couple of minutes, merges with the yellow-blazed Hoeferlin Trail (HT). Continue straight, now guided by yellow and blue tree tags.

The rubble-strewn track staggers north-northwest, delivering an oak- and laurel-filtered glimpse of Ramapo Lake. Hang with the MT as it shifts left among a thicket of blueberry bushes, and make a left, once it descends to pavement, toward the water. Then, in something like 15 paces, roll right, remaining on the pavement and still with blue blazes (diverging from the yellow markings). Now shuffling counterclockwise around the rock-studded shore of the lake, enjoy the view across its lily pad–speckled surface, with a craggy escarpment on your right.

To continue with the circuit, bear left at the fork at the northwest corner of the lake, even as the MT breaks away and forges uphill along the old estate road. Ramapo Lake, by the way, lies over a glacial depression formed during the last ice age, around 13,000 years ago. For secluded access to the lake, take the gravel-surfaced spur that appears in a couple of minutes on the left. It leads to an oak-shaded nook where you can enjoy a quiet moment by the water before proceeding with the remainder of the hike.

Back on the main trail, go left (south), and hold to the left in about 30 paces, as the Cannonball Trail (CT, marked by a white C on red) merges from the right. Remain with the CT all the way to the south end of the lake, turning left at the slanted T where it breaks to the right. Your time on this level, unblazed forest road ends at the next junction, which appears in 35 yards, at which point take a right, leaving the lakeshore vicinity. This wide track gently ascends for a moment before steadily losing elevation. Remain straight when the HT rejoins your route from the right (it connects with the CT), its yellow blazes now coloring the trees. A few minutes later, the HT breaks left, on a narrower spur; follow it (and the yellow blazes), departing the main track.

Stick with the HT as it jumps left again, in roughly ten strides, while the noise of interstate-highway traffic begins to penetrate the tree cover. That sound escalates from a dull roar to deafening thunder as you stagger onward an additional 25 yards to the next fork. Your circuit breaks left there, but take a moment, if your ears can endure the cacophony, to venture to the right, on a spur that leads (once you pass through a hole in a chain-link fence and swing left at the T), to an eagle's-nest overlook of I-287. This remarkably fine view is a fair trade-off for the head-pounding sound of steady traffic. When you tire of this setting, return to the main trail and bear right, back on the HT.

There are a few more vistas of I-287, filtered through the forest, as the HT zigzags downhill and bypasses a wide spur on the right. The single-file path finally pulls free of the highway noise while hugging the granite-studded hillside. In five to eight minutes of scrambling over grass and lichen-speckled bedrock, you should reach the crest, at 711 feet. Just beyond the clutch of pitch pines, by the slanted slab of granite, the red-blazed Lookout Trail merges with the HT. Go left here, on a very pleasant stretch now marked with both yellow and red blazes.

A few rocky patches ensue, among tangled clusters of mountain laurel. Once you've threaded your way through this stretch and clawed to the top of a rocky knob where birch trees, scrub oaks, and pitch pines encircle the scene, you'll be rewarded with a fine view of Ramapo Lake. A pleasant sun-exposed stroll among calf-high blueberry bushes succeeds this, as you meander along the spine of the ridge. And then—just like that—the HT pops out of the forest to join the wide lakeside circuit as the red blazes end.

Swing right on the gravel-surfaced lane and proceed directly toward the dam. Ignore the red-blazed route on the right—that's the other end of the horseshoe-shaped Lookout Trail—and cross over the concrete barrier, bearing right when you reach the roadway. Almost immediately, within 15 paces, the blue-blazed MacEvoy bolts into the woods to the right, leading you back to the trailhead.

■ TO THE TRAILHEAD

Take Exit 57 off I-287 onto Skyline Drive, Ringwood direction. In 0.1 mile, turn left into the parking lot.

20 Watchung Sierra Sampler

■ OVERVIEW

LENGTH: 5.7 miles	**ACCESS:** Year-round, dawn–dusk; no fee; pets must be leashed
CONFIGURATION: Loop	**MAPS:** At visitor center; USGS Chatham
SCENERY: Gently rolling terrain boasts mixed forests, a placid lake, several bogs, an abandoned village, and some exceptionally tall tulip trees	**FACILITIES:** None along trail, but visitor center has restrooms, water, and a public phone; park offers picnic areas, a playground, and a campground
EXPOSURE: Semi-shady	
TRAIL SURFACE: Dirt, roots, rocks	**COMMENTS:** In springtime, the dogwoods and rhododendrons flower abundantly. For general information, call (908) 527-4900, or visit www.union countynj.org/parks/wrmap804.pdf.
TRAFFIC: Can get really heavy on summer weekends	
HIKING TIME: 3 hours	

■ SNAPSHOT

With several miles of trails, you have are plenty of opportunities to lose yourself among the hardwoods and conifers that color so much of this county park. A couple of ponds, a long, narrow lake (where oddly shaped erratics decorate its shoreline), and the well-preserved remnants of a mill town–cum–resort community contribute to the delights of the hike. Other highlights include the diverse bird populations that thrive around water holes, and herds of deer that chomp through the woods.

■ CLOSEUP

Gesundheit! That, in a word, is the response we hear most often on bringing Watchung into a conversation. In fact, *Watchung* is actually a corruption of *wachunk,* a Lenape Indian word for "high hills," and there are two soaring ridges of the Watchung Mountains running the length of the park, with a bubbling brook and Lake Surprise nestled in between. Watchung also

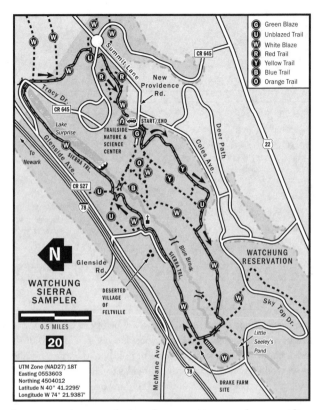

WATCHUNG SIERRA SAMPLER

20

Green Blaze
Unblazed Trail
White Blaze
Red Trail
Yellow Trail
Blue Trail
Orange Trail

0.5 MILES

UTM Zone (NAD27) 18T
Easting 0553603
Northing 4504012
Latitude N 40° 41.2295'
Longitude W 74° 21.9387'

features a playground, greenhouse, various gardens, a riding stable, ball fields, a scout camp, a picnic area, a trailside museum, a planetarium—even the well-preserved buildings of a 19th-century company town.

Considering all that, the hiking in Watchung is pretty darn good. An intricate network of trails covers much of the reservation's 2,000 acres, with the white-blazed Sierra Trail (ST) circling the perimeter for a total of 10 miles. The following trek overlaps a large segment of the ST, providing a fine introduction to the largest preserve in Union County.

Start at the southwest corner of the parking lot, and stride west over the paved road to the archway entrance of the Nature Trail. The path, blazed with both green and white swatches, descends to a bridge, then cuts upward by a bench and a couple of birdhouses. Two more seasonal streams follow, as well as some ups and downs. Take the yellow-blazed spur that appears on the left, gaining ground and meandering into an overgrown forest of maples, oaks, and tulip trees.

Leave this yellow path in roughly five minutes for the unblazed stem slightly to the left. Ignore the side traces and increase your pace as this route brushes against a residential neighborhood, picking up such native noises as barking dogs and lawn mowers. Swing left at the T, following the white blazes of the ST. Swerve left again when the ST collides with a bridle path.

In less than a minute, the level, dirt-surfaced trail meets another junction. Go right, toward Blue Brook, on the unmarked gravel path, as the ST veers left. Hop over the bridge and press onward, bypassing the left toward a boardwalk and Little Seeley's Pond. The next right is yours, a continuation of the ST as it now travels northeastward, into a somewhat wilder stretch of trail. Don't be drawn off the ST by the many side trails; the Deserted Village of Feltville lies directly ahead.

No, that's not the title of a new Stephen King novel. Feltville originated as a company mill town in 1845, was later converted to a resort community, and eventually abandoned; in 1980 the site was placed on the National Register of Historic Places. Off-white with green trim, the houses seem invitingly intact and well maintained. Look more closely, though, and aside from three that are still inhabited, most are in various stages of decay. Stick with the paved road as it leads from Masker's Barn past three houses and a trail to the right. (Keep an eye out for white-tailed deer, which often graze in the area.) Another pair of houses follows; then, as the road bends leftward, there is a turnoff to the right for the cemetery, where the pavement reaches the old church and store. Go with that spur, on the near side of the church, to the pocket graveyard. Contrary to what the five headstones suggest, the small fenced plot is believed to hold something like two dozen bodies. The only original stone is on the far right, and supposedly none of them mark the correct grave. Maybe there's a Stephen King story here after all.

Pick up the white blazes of the ST at the front of the cemetery, where the trail nudges northeast back into the forest. Bear left at the fork, then make a right at the T, joining a wide bridle path; as the trail arcs downhill, follow the white markings to the left; scuttle right in another eight steps onto the narrow conduit between two towering tulip trees. This lush, grassy setting gives way to Lake Surprise, where large erratics populate its shore.

As you walk clockwise around the lake, the Sierra and bridle path briefly kiss, then diverge again, with your route running to the right. Now it gets tricky. On reaching County Road 645, keep to the right shoulder, pass over the bridge, and then cross to the left side of the road. Bear left on the cinder driveway, just a few paces beyond the bridge; then turn right at the first intersection, momentarily leaving the ST. Skip the spur 30 yards ahead; the ST reunites with the track from the direction of the stables but sheers off to the left near the road, one minute after you pass a wide bridle path on the left. Steer to the right on the cinder track, cross the road, then make a left at the first fork and a right at the second, as the white blazes once more join the path. Remain with the ST all the way back to the parking lot.

■ TO THE TRAILHEAD

From I-78 west, take Exit 43 and merge right onto Diamond Hill Road. Go right at the traffic light, onto McMane Avenue. At the next traffic light, turn left onto Glenside Avenue, and in 1.4 miles hang a right to enter the reservation. Proceed past Lake Surprise to the traffic circle, taking the first right, Summit Lane, and in 0.4 miles go right again on New Providence Road, which leads in 0.2 miles to the trailhead on the left, across from the Trailside Nature & Science Center parking lot and the nearby visitor center.